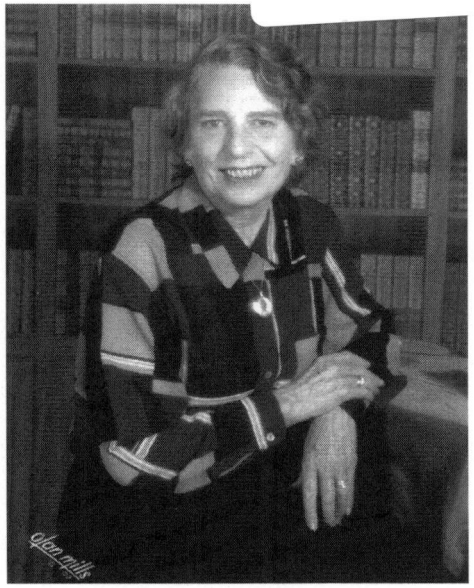

Marian Tidswell MA, FCSP, Dip TP, ONC
Photo by Olan Mills

MARIAN TIDSWELL is an orthopaedic nurse and physiotherapist and worked as a physiotherapist and aftercare sister prior to gaining teaching qualifications. She joined the staff at Oswestry and North Staffordshire School of Physiotherapy in 1968, first as a teacher, then principal.

In retirement, she remains actively involved with the profession.

ADVERSITY THE SPUR

*THE HISTORY OF
PHYSIOTHERAPY EDUCATION
AT OSWESTRY*

ADVERSITY THE SPUR

THE HISTORY OF PHYSIOTHERAPY EDUCATION AT OSWESTRY

MARIAN TIDSWELL

ATHENA PRESS
LONDON

ADVERSITY THE SPUR
The History of Physiotherapy Education at Oswestry
Copyright © Marian Tidswell 2009

All Rights Reserved

No part of this book may be reproduced in any form
by photocopying or by any electronic or mechanical means,
including information storage or retrieval systems,
without permission in writing from both the copyright
owner and the publisher of this book.

ISBN 978 1 84748 522 9

First published 2009 by
ATHENA PRESS
Queen's House, 2 Holly Road
Twickenham TW1 4EG
United Kingdom

Printed for Athena Press

Acknowledgements

At some point during the late 1980s, Mary Powell, the last matron of the Robert Jones and Agnes Hunt Orthopaedic Hospital, who is also a qualified chartered physiotherapist, suggested that the many changes with which the school at Oswestry was currently involved should be chronicled. The school was at the time embroiled in the turmoil of radical change arising from alterations in course operation demanded by the Chartered Society of Physiotherapy and the proposals for rationalisation of physiotherapy education in the West Midlands Regional Health Authority. When in a position to undertake the task following retirement, many people gave support to the venture, notably my husband John, whose consistent encouragement throughout the protracted period of manuscript preparation has been invaluable.

The chief executive of the Robert Jones and Agnes Hunt Orthopaedic and District Hospital Trust approved the project and the Education Department of the Chartered Society of Physiotherapy permitted access to minutes of the Education Committee pertaining to the school.

Many former students supplied reminiscences and memories of their time at Oswestry. Those who qualified more recently supplied verbal information, whereas those who trained at an earlier time provided written comments, copies of relevant articles and photographs to substantiate the text. A group reminiscence by students who undertook the physiotherapy course between 1959 and 1962 was gratefully received and comprehensive individual contributions were received from Hazel Roberts, Audrey Alexander, Nora Orritt, Mary Gardner and Betty Linklater, who all studied at the hospital between 1943 and 1948. K.E. Rowe and Mary Powell, who trained between 1936 and 1941, also made helpful contributions, as did Edna Longson, who trained with Sister Arthur between 1923 and 1927. Edna lived until 29 February 2008, when she died at the age of 102. The earliest contributions from two Baschurch trainees, Peggy Lovatt (1916–1919) and Dr Frances Taylor (1914–1917), were supplied by Marie Carter, the health sciences librarian at the Institute of Orthopaedics at the Robert Jones and Agnes Hunt Orthopaedic Hospital.

Marie Carter permitted me access to minutes, annual reports, nursing notes and other documentation from the earliest days of the hospital and to the *Journal of the Old Oswestrian Physiotherapists Association*, published in the late 1950s. The third edition of *The Heritage of Oswestry* by Douglas Cruttenden, *Healing & Hope* by Marie Carter, and *This is My Life* by Agnes Hunt provided further insight to the origins and development of the school.

The support and encouragement willingly given by the Old Oswestrian Physiotherapists Association, the Robert Jones and Agnes Hunt Orthopaedic and District NHS Trust, the Chartered Society of Physiotherapy, Mary Powell and former students, family and friends who have read and commented on selected chapters of the text is gratefully acknowledged. The most consistent encouragement and the most valuable comments have been received from Marie Carter, without whom the book would not have been completed.

I am most grateful to all who have been involved for enabling me to complete the text.

Preface

The majority of physiotherapists currently in practice in the UK are graduate entrants to the profession. They are competent and confident within their field of expertise and are guardians of the unique body of knowledge known as physiotherapy. They work within a framework guided by a strict code of professional practice and ethical by-laws.

A mere thirty years ago, all qualifying physiotherapists on the UK mainland entered the profession having followed hospital-based courses that granted them eligibility for membership of the Chartered Society of Physiotherapy. The Chartered Society is the professional organisation for physiotherapists which, at that time, set, examined and monitored the majority of physiotherapy pre-qualification courses. The courses had no educational recognition or rating and qualified practitioners treated patients that had been referred by doctors, dentists or veterinary surgeons. The situation changed completely over the two decades from the mid seventies to the mid nineties.

Prior to the introduction of the NHS, there were approximately thirty-five courses in the UK, the majority of which were based in general hospitals. They were small, each course having a total student body that numbered between sixty and one hundred with approximately 1,000 new registrants entering the profession annually. Schools tended to be educationally isolated and, although following the nationally determined curriculum, developed individual characteristics that made them recognisable one from the other. These could be related to the range and quality of the clinical education available or the amount of access to university departments for particular aspects of the course. It is apparent that people tend to recruit in their own image and much of the individuality identified between schools could be traced to this situation.

When the NHS was introduced in 1948, it retained financial

control and overall responsibility for the education and training of certain paramedical groups including physiotherapy, when it had been an obvious opportunity to transfer the courses to the higher education sector. The NHS was concerned primarily with training a workforce to satisfy treatment needs of patients at minimal cost to the service. It had neither the resources nor the inclination to enhance the qualification of these groups beyond the competencies required by practitioners to fulfil this role. Although the monies for the training of doctors and nurses were ring-fenced from the point of allocation to the point of usage, no such arrangement existed for physiotherapy training budgets. Once allocated centrally, these monies were not recognisable in the overall subregional allocated budgets to health authorities. The lack of ring-fencing enabled hard-pressed hospital management teams to 'borrow' varying proportions of these annual financial training allocations to achieve specific targets in other areas of individual health authority responsibility, often to improve specific aspects of direct patient care.

One of the oldest schools of physiotherapy that now operates from a university base is the one founded at Baschurch in Shropshire in 1909 by Dame Agnes Hunt. She was a charismatic person who defied family, social convention and significant physical disability to devote her life to the service of people with orthopaedic problems. After a strenuous career in district nursing, she established a small convalescent home in a house on the family estate in Baschurch and it was here that the school of physiotherapy, which is the subject of this book, was founded. She developed the physical treatment of patients with orthopaedic disability and has been identified as the Florence Nightingale of orthopaedics. In subsequent partnership with a pioneering orthopaedic surgeon, she developed the hospital that now bears their names. Without her background and experience with pain and physical disability, and her conviction that disabled people could make a valuable contribution to the workforce, it is unlikely that the hospital, school of physiotherapy or the Derwen Cripples Training College at Gobowen would have been established. Throughout its long history, qualifiers from Oswestry retained many of the characteristics of the founder. As practitioners they are recognised for their sound clinical skills; they have determination and persistence bordering on obstinacy and the ability to cope calmly with challenging situations. They have a strong sense of justice, and are devoted to their profession and loyal to their training school.

As educational opportunities expanded for many occupations during the fifties and sixties, educational development of the paramedical professions was inhibited due to the funding basis in health rather than education. Health authorities supporting schools of physiotherapy found that degree courses were, in the main, too expensive to implement and maintain, and in most cases were not in a position to support degree course development. Physiotherapy training courses remained without educational recognition until the Open University assessed the curriculum and recognised the courses to be at diploma level, equivalent to two years' full-time study in tertiary education. Gaining this educational rating was a significant step in the profession's development.

During the 1990s, changes in the number and distribution of training schools and alteration of the funding base for education and training from district to regional health authority control facilitated the achievement of graduate entry in 1994. The decision to pursue this course of action had been taken some fourteen years earlier by the CSP Education Committee and endorsed by its council. Its achievement in so short a timescale resulted from persistent campaigning, the educational rating given by the Open University and significant changes in the management and financing of the initial education of physiotherapists. Physiotherapy as a profession has benefited significantly from assimilation into the academic environment, as its research base is now being developed and individual expertise is recognised by the formation of clinical specialist and extended-scope practitioner posts.

While in the throes of the changes occurring in physiotherapy education during the 1980s, the need to document the process became apparent to ensure future graduates remained cognisant of the origins and development of their profession. The Oswestry and North Staffordshire School of Physiotherapy was an obvious subject for this consideration as it was unusually based in a specialist hospital and was, uniquely, funded by not one but two health authorities.

The title of this book, *Adversity the Spur*, is taken from D.I. Cruttenden's preface to the third edition of *The Heritage of Oswestry* which bears the subtitle 'The Origin and Development of the Robert Jones and Agnes Hunt Orthopaedic Hospital 1900–1975'. The context in which the phrase appears identifies the sense of this centre of orthopaedic excellence and is quoted here.

> The contribution of many hundreds of good people who gave freely of their time, energy and thought in the voluntary work for the well-being of the Hospital and its patients has been of incalculable value and encouragement to those whose chosen task was to heal, to care for and to rehabilitate the disabled and to those who chose to teach and to seek for progress through research.
>
> The Oswestry 'family' is justly proud of its heritage and in all humility may claim to have preserved and perpetuated the Spirit of Oswestry handed down from the past.
>
> This 'Spirit' is no ephemeral fancy, it is an intangible amalgam of team work, skills of a high order, youthful exuberance and confidence, courage to express new ideas, wisdom to listen and learn from others with different experience, and above all human kindness and consideration for others and a cheerful optimistic approach to any problem, dedicated to the needs of the disabled. It pervades the whole staff and those who serve voluntarily.
>
> It was a great privilege to have been associated with this happy and enthusiastic team to whom adversity was the spur, as it was to Dame Agnes, and with whom I learned the value of the human touch, of good humour in times of difficulty and of determination.

The school changed its name several times during its existence as it adjusted to new criteria and faced different challenges and is now firmly established in Keele University. The long and sometimes arduous journey from Baschurch to Keele is charted in this text, which accounts the progress of the school from its origins in a small private specialist hospital to becoming part of a thriving university. The school reaches its centenary in October

2009 and the story of its progress from 1909 to 1996 is the period covered by this text.

To encourage factual accuracy, extensive use has been made of minutes of the various committees supporting the school during its long life and also reports and other information sources available to the school. The author takes responsibility for any inaccuracies that inadvertently have been presented in the text and apologises for them in advance.

KEY DATES IN SCHOOL HISTORY

- 1900 The Baschurch Convalescent Home opened.
- 1904 Surgery commenced at the Baschurch Convalescent Home and Hospital.
- 1908 Course in orthopaedic nursing started for lady pupil probationers who received no salary and provided their own uniforms.
- 1909 Approval granted to train students in massage and Swedish remedial exercise with the Incorporated Society of Trained Masseuses – ISTMS.
- 1909 School of Massage started at Stoke-on-Trent with the Northern Guild of Massage. Closed after five years.
- 1911 Three students entered for ISTMS examinations.
- 1919 One of the 1911 qualifiers started the School of Massage at the Manchester Royal Infirmary.
- 1920 Royal Charter granted to ISTMS which also merged with the Institute of Massage and Medical Gymnastics to become the Chartered Society of Massage and Medical Gymnastics (CSMMG).
- 1921 Transfer of the hospital to Gobowen, now called the Shropshire Orthopaedic Hospital.
- 1922 New massage department opened with three staff and eleven students.
- 1923 Miss Dalton appointed in August to be principal of the Oswestry School of Physiotherapy.

1943 Society renamed Chartered Society of Physiotherapy (CSP).

1945 Miss Dorothy Talbot appointed principal of the Oswestry School of Physiotherapy.

1948 Fire destroyed several wards and the physiotherapy department.

1952 New School of Physiotherapy opened on the floor above the physiotherapy department. It had two lecture rooms, a practical classroom and a clinical laboratory.

1967 Appointment of Miss M.I. Anderson as first principal of the Oswestry and North Staffordshire School of Physiotherapy (ONSSP).

1969 Oswestry and North Staffordshire School of Physiotherapy (ONSSP) established.

1974 Miss Wyn Cannell appointed principal of ONSSP.

1975 New CSP course established.

1981 Mrs Marian Tidswell appointed principal of ONSSP. First male students enrolled on course.

1988 Last intake to study for the Charted Society of Physiotherapy course and national examinations.

1989 First intake to the Graduate Diploma Course with internal assessment.

1991 BSc (Hons) validated as an external degree of Keele University. First cohort completed the course from the hospital base.

1992 First cohort from ONSSP to have completed the Graduate Diploma in Physiotherapy with internalised assessment.

1993 Mrs Marian Tidswell appointed head of the department of physiotherapy studies of Keele University.

1994 Graduate entry to physiotherapy achieved in the United Kingdom. First cohort to graduate from the Oswestry and North Staffordshire School of Physiotherapy/Keele University.

1995 Second BSc (Hons) Physiotherapy course validated. Faculty of Health (initially called D Board) established at Keele University. Marian Tidswell elected to be first deputy dean of the faculty.

1996 Mrs Marilyn Place appointed head of department of physiotherapy studies.

Contents

Chapter 1
One Spring Afternoon — 19

Chapter 2
The Early Years: 1867–1900 — 21

Chapter 3
Baschurch Convalescent Home: 1900–1909 — 32

Chapter 4
Early Years of the School of Massage: 1909–1920 — 42

Chapter 5
The School of Physiotherapy at Oswestry: 1920–1945 — 53

Chapter 6
Preparing for the National Health Service: 1942–1948 — 73

Chapter 7
A Year of Change: 1948 — 84

Chapter 8
Course Affiliation – Wolverhampton: 1948–1957 — 92

Chapter 9
Affiliation with the Royal Salop Infirmary: 1957–1969 — 108

Chapter 10
The Oswestry and North Staffordshire School of
Physiotherapy: 1969–1974 — 128

Chapter 11
The Oswestry and North Staffordshire School of
Physiotherapy: 1974–1981   146

Chapter 12
A Time of Renewal: 1981–1983   168

Chapter 13
Upgrading and Course Development: 1984–1986   190

Chapter 14
Regional Training Council Activity: 1987   210

Illustrations   between 228 and 229

Chapter 15
Course Internalisation: 1988 Onwards   229

Chapter 16
BSc (Honours) Physiotherapy   249

Chapter 17
Rationalisation of Schools of Physiotherapy in the
West Midlands Region   269

Chapter 18
A New Beginning   286

Bibliography   298

Index   303

Chapter 1
One Spring Afternoon

She was seen entering the garden moving slowly into the sunlight. A person of average height, she appeared to be in her early forties, dressed in a simple practical style, wearing a dress of neutral colour, a form of head covering and a long apron. She seemed distracted, possibly worried, but certainly oblivious to her surroundings.

It was a warm, slightly overcast day in May 1909 in the Shropshire village of Baschurch. At Florence House, the early spring flowers had given way to patches of bluebells clumped around the roots of the mature trees dotted around the property. Lilac, hawthorn, cherry and blackthorn blossom added further colour and lightly perfumed the air. The chirruping bickering of hungry fledglings mingled with muted clangings, chattering and laughter drifting across the lawn from the house and the buildings scattered about the large garden.

As she entered the garden, an area of comparative peace and tranquillity, she was obviously appreciative of the familiar, relaxed atmosphere in which she was enveloped. She was, however, somewhat at odds with the lighthearted cheerfulness around her. As she walked slowly across the lawn, she pondered the latest of the many problems that had beset the hospital that occupied both the house she had just left and the buildings scattered around the garden. This place was more than just her place of work, more than just her home; it was her life. It was here that she had taken her first uncertain steps towards the fulfilment of an incredible dream that had dominated her life. In this place, she had begun to satisfy ideals she had held for more than thirty years.

Agnes – for this was her name – sought a few moments' solitude. She needed to distance herself from the clamour of the wards, her mother's peremptory demands and the unending pressures and responsibilities that battled for supremacy in her mind as she went about her professional duties in this quiet corner of England. The particular problem presently dominating her thoughts had been developing over the last two or three years, but had now reached crisis level – a solution had to be found if the hospital was to survive and she was to fulfil her destiny.

She walked hesitantly, deep in thought, across the three quarters of an acre of the garden that spread out and around her, moving towards the open-sided sheds at the lower end of the property. Pausing occasionally, she leaned heavily on her crutch and eased the weight off her right foot. She longed for relief from the intense pain that constantly emanated from her right hip and cursed the high atmospheric humidity, so often a feature of Shropshire weather, as it contributed significantly to her overall discomfort, limited her physical activities and reduced her capacity for clarity of thought.

After some minutes in deep contemplation, her attitude seemed to have changed. As she raised her head, one could see a cautious smile had replaced the furrows of concentration on her brow. She seemed to gain in stature and appeared lighter of spirit as she turned and, in a purposeful manner, headed back toward the house. The pain and disablement, so long a major part of her life, temporarily faded into insignificance, where she firmly believed it belonged. An idea was germinating in her mind that could provide a solution to the immediate problem.

She hurried, retracing her steps to the house, in search of her friend and co-founder of the hospital, Emily Goodford, with whom all matters of importance were discussed fully before any action was taken. In this instance, it was hoped the idea that had come to Agnes during her walk in the garden would be capable of development into a sound plan which could prove to be the salvation of the hospital.

Chapter 2
The Early Years: 1867–1900

The nineteenth century as portrayed by literature and historical record shows considerable disparity of provision and expectations between the 'rich' and 'poor'. On the one hand there was comfort, carefree elegance and culture, on the other poverty, illiteracy and despair. Families in comfortable financial situations employed many servants to care for their needs and these, in turn, were then able to support their own families. Being born into wealth and privilege also brought obligations to help all the less financially secure families living on their estates. The wives and daughters of the estate-owning family regularly visited these less fortunate households and provided additional food or clothing, particularly to help them survive the long winter months. England was still largely an agrarian-based society with the advantages and disadvantages of the final years of a social structure that retained many elements of feudalism.

There was, at this time, considerable unrest among the lower income groups in rural areas. The unending supply of labour required to operate machinery in the wake of the Industrial Revolution encouraged the employed workers to leave the countryside in droves, seeking promised wealth and opportunity offered by new technologies. The reality was less congenial than the anticipation, as the move to industrial areas led to rapid population growth around the new factories, producing intense overcrowding. The work offered was underpaid and arduous, and all that the charitable support workers had enjoyed in the country was now denied. Slums developed in most of these new urban development areas where disease was rife, despair and violence the norm, and grinding poverty was all that many of the population could anticipate before their blessed release by an early death.

Impoverished workers fell into the clutches of greedy slum landlords who charged extortionate rents for very poor housing. Rental of one of these hovels took most of a worker's wages. Any remaining money was used to buy food, but there was never enough to satisfy the needs of the family. Wives and children of the poor slum dwellers would scavenge through rubbish bins in the hopes of finding something eatable among festering piles of rotting fruit and vegetables. Thus a large section of the population constantly struggled to make ends meet. Maternal mortality was high and many babies were stillborn while others lived days or weeks only. For the survivors, work by the age of six or seven was the norm. Although their labour was extremely poorly recompensed, if they were healthy, they made some contribution to the family income and paid for their share of the frugal nourishment available.

For a child born with, for example, a twisted foot or a curved spine, the future was even more uncertain. Physical deformity of this type was not life-threatening; therefore the meagre family resources would not be used to pay for medical care. If the child survived infancy, the untreated deformity would exaggerate with growth and subsequently exclude the afflicted person from employment. Children in this situation were unable to make any financial contribution to the family income. Once their continuing wants and needs could no longer be satisfied, many were neglected and slowly starved to death, while others were thrown out of their homes and took to the streets where they scratched a living by begging or stealing. The slums were teeming with these outcasts of society, cripples of all ages who had forgotten their past and had no hope for the future.

These were the times into which Agnes was born and lived her early life. Rowland Hunt, her father, was born in 1829, eight years before Victoria came to the British throne and eighty years before Agnes was found walking in the Baschurch garden. Rowland was destined to become the head of a long-established Shropshire landowning family. His wife, Florence Marianne Humfrey, a wealthy heiress with estates in Leicestershire and Northamptonshire, possessed boundless energy and enthusiasm. She was a very capable organiser and charity fundraiser, and was also an accomplished hostess with a wide circle of friends. These talents and experience were to be put to good use in her later life. Between the ages of twenty-one and forty, she produced eleven children, all of whom survived to adulthood. Her sixth child, Agnes Gwendoline, born on 31 December 1867, commented in her autobiography that her mother disliked children when they were coming, during their arrival and most intensely after they had arrived,[1] a factor that had considerable influence on their childhood and upbringing. Florence Marianne was also a very determined woman of whom Agnes said, on one occasion, that you might as well try to stop the Niagara Falls as stop her mother when she had made up her mind.[2] She was regarded with awe and respect by her numerous children, who soon learned the safest route through childhood was to keep out of her way whenever possible.

The children were all subjected to harsh parental discipline with enthusiastic adherence to the Victorian ideal of corporal punishment as the prime instrument of behaviour regulation. In this environment, very strong inter-sibling bonds of loyalty and fortitude developed which were to last throughout their lives.

With their parents absent for much of the time, responsibility for the children's daily care was delegated to a children's nurse they adored and a series of governesses they terrified.[3] Although Mrs Hunt had the minimum of direct contact with her children as befitted her position in mid-Victorian society, she had very strong ideas about their upbringing, believing implicitly in the positive benefits of fresh air and exercise. The children lived on and had the freedom of the large Boreatton Park estate, part of the Hunt family lands in Shropshire, where they spent most of their free time playing energetic games that were the product of their uninhibited imaginations. Even with harsh discipline and the distant relationship with their parents, childhood memories are recalled with humour and pleasure by Dame Agnes and, despite the worst prognostications of one despairing governess who was surprised by the number of innovative ways the children had discovered by which to kill themselves,[4] all survived to adulthood.

This comfortable, carefree life was irretrievably changed for Agnes when, at nine years of age, she developed a high fever and severe pain in her right hip. As her mother did not accept that there was any such thing as illness,[5] Agnes endeavoured to disguise her pain. She was able to hide her distress for a number of days, suffering stoically in silence and trying to behave in as normal a manner as possible so she would not draw attention to herself and risk incurring the wrath of her parents. However, her reaction to a friendly pat on the shoulder by an adult visitor was so violent that the family realised she had a significant problem and, immediately, all resources available at the time were directed towards her care.

Mrs Hunt was devastated. Having raised eleven healthy, lively children safely through the dangerous early years of childhood, she was forced to accept that one, at the age of nine, was now critically ill. It is difficult to imagine nowadays a child with septic arthritis of the hip not being treated successfully; however, in the late 1870s, without modern-day technical knowledge, diagnostic aids and appropriate medication for the majority of conditions, being ill was always a life-threatening and often a terminal situation.

Fortunately, her parents did not consider hospital treatment, where Agnes would probably have been subjected to a procedure performed by a surgeon wearing soiled clothes that were stiff with patients' blood from previous operations. As anaesthetics and antiseptic procedures were not in universal use, the surgery would have been performed with unsterilised instruments, possibly without anaesthetic and, if she survived the shock of the operation, she would undoubtedly have succumbed to post-operative infection. Hospital buildings were ill-equipped, dirty, overcrowded, teeming with infection and, worse, there was no routine nursing care for the sick. For these reasons, sick people generally had a far better chance of recovery if nursed at home away from the contaminants of the hospital environment.

This, fortunately, was how her problem was managed and Agnes was cared for at home by the family's children's nurse. Her early childhood, with its emphasis on outdoor activities and fresh air, combined with the healthy diet enjoyed by all the family, had enabled her to develop the strong constitution and strength of character required to withstand and eventually overcome the infection that had overwhelmed her small frame. Once she had overcome the infection, it was apparent that, although she would be restored to full general health, she would have residual scarring in the hip which would leave her with limited movement and a deformity that would increase with growth. It was at this point the full implications of the illness became apparent to the family – Agnes was now a cripple. Her life, and that of her family, was permanently altered.

Mrs Hunt was no ordinary person and did not follow the traditional response to the situation, a factor that shaped Agnes's future life as much as the illness that had almost ended it. As Agnes regained her strength, although undeniably crippled by the septic arthritis, she was encouraged to behave as an able-bodied child. Her brothers and sisters were forbidden to make any concessions for her reduced physical capabilities or to give her any obvious assistance. She had started her 'apprenticeship to crippledom and the great education of pain'.[6] Thus she remained a lively member of the outdoor culture instilled in the family from early childhood. For example, during the winter she would be strapped to a sledge and made to keep goal for the impromptu family games of ice hockey. During the summer months, her bath chair was often to be seen harnessed to the family pony and used by all the children as a racing vehicle.[7]

Without antibiotics or other significant effective medication, Agnes's disabling hip condition recurred frequently and, in later years, she was constantly in pain and seldom seen without sticks or crutches. At all times she participated fully in family and social activities and was not encouraged or allowed to retire into obscurity and assume Victorian society's conventional image of a cripple.

Unfortunately, the family's settled life was further shattered and permanently altered in 1879, when Agnes was twelve, by the unexpected death of her fifty-year-old father. A businessman who spent much of his time away from home, he was in many ways a distant figure to his family, but his death had far-reaching effects on their lives. Devastated by her husband's death, Florence Marianne Hunt lost focus and eventually left Boreatton Hall to return to her Leicestershire estate, prior to a five-year spell in

Australia and Tasmania with Agnes and her younger brothers and sisters. This time in Australia was physically very arduous for all the family and, while there, Agnes suffered several exacerbations of her hip problem which she survived despite lack of adequate medical or nursing care during the acute, life-threatening phases of the disease. The family eventually drifted back to England with Agnes arriving in London in April 1887. Partly as a result of her experiences of illness while abroad, she returned to England with the intention of training as a nurse.[8]

Although one could not deny Agnes was, by this time, significantly disabled, she had already proved, with her mother's help, that a crippled person could lead a normal active life. She had sufficient personal income to obviate the necessity for employment and, whatever plans Mrs Hunt had for her daughter's future, nursing was not one of the options she would consider. To seek employment in a hospital was inappropriate to the family's social standing. Mrs Hunt vigorously opposed Agnes's choice of career as she considered it demeaning and degrading, and she also considered that no daughter of hers would have the courage to complete the training course.[9]

For some time, there were discussions, debates and disputes between the spirited mother and the daughter who had inherited all her mother's determination. After several months Agnes finally overcame her mother's strong resistance to the proposal and received her reluctant consent. To her credit, having finally given permission for Agnes to train as a nurse, Mrs Hunt supported and encouraged her with as much enthusiasm as she had previously expended on opposing such an unexpected choice.

Once she had obtained maternal approval, Agnes applied to hospitals for acceptance as a probationer nurse or a lady pupil. The main difference between these routes to qualification was that the probationer nurse training lasted for two years before the award of the certificate and tuition was free, whereas the lady pupil training course for nurses was completed in a year, but a fee was charged for tuition. Initially Agnes's applications for either option were rejected on the grounds that she was too young and too lame to train as a nurse, and she failed to gain a place in any London teaching hospital.[10]

Her perseverance and determination were rewarded eventually when she was accepted as a lady pupil at the Royal Alexandra Hospital in Rhyl, a hospital that catered mainly for crippled children and that advocated fresh air and happiness as essential components of all treatment regimes.

Before her year's training was completed, Agnes transferred to the West London Hospital, Hammersmith, in order to gain more experience in general nursing. This hospital had not yet adopted Miss Nightingale's principles of organisation or nursing practice and exemplified many of the worst characteristics of nineteenth-century hospital life. The nurses' food was insufficient and unappetising, and the work far too hard for young trainees. The duty shift was twelve hours long with the possibility of two hours' break every second day. This rest depended on the numbers of staff fit enough to work. It is hard to say who was more at risk – patients who had survived surgery or the nursing staff employed to give them post-operative care. Agnes managed three months in this inhospitable environment before collapsing with exhaustion, and determined at that point that, if she were to complete her training and to work in nursing, she would not subject her staff to such drudgery as she had experienced at the West London Hospital. After six weeks' rest and recuperation, she transferred to the Salop Infirmary at Shrewsbury where she finally gained her certificate of qualification in 1891.[11]

As soon as she achieved full nurse status, Agnes embarked on a six-month course in district nursing to qualify as a Queens Nurse. It was during this part of her training that she met with Emily Goodford. Despite an age difference of ten years, Agnes and Emily became very close friends, working together for almost three decades until Emily's untimely death in February 1920. Agnes completed her nurse education by training as a midwife and, over the next few years, took a six-month post as midwife on the Isle of Wight followed by about two years in Rushden, fighting a typhoid epidemic. Late in 1894, she and Emily moved to Middlesbrough to help nurse victims of a smallpox epidemic and after this were employed as district nurses based in Ollerton in North Yorkshire.[12]

About the same time as Agnes Hunt and Emily Goodford

were heading towards Middlesbrough, four young nurses from the London Hospital, who were also properly trained in massage and 'medical rubbing', determined to form a society of massage. They were very concerned by the activities of untrained practitioners and by the numerous articles that had appeared in the *British Medical Journal* and the *Lancet* warning doctors against the use of massage techniques to treat patients owing to the number of untrained, unscrupulous practitioners offering their services.[13] The purpose of this society was threefold: 'to protect legitimate practitioners from the slurs prevalent at the time', to 'restore the good name of massage treatment for the sick and injured' and finally, to 'make massage a safe, clean and honourable profession for British women'.[14]

The Society of Trained Masseuses (STM) was formed late in 1894 by these four nurses: Lucy Marianne Robinson, Rosalind Paget, Elizabeth Anne Manley and Margaret Dora Palmer. By the following year, membership of the society had expanded to such an extent that they were able to elect a council of nine from their membership, to regulate the society's affairs.[15] They also established regular examinations in massage techniques with the award of certificates to successful candidates. By these means a standard of professional knowledge and competence of practitioner members of the society was determined and, for their individual protection, Rules of Professional Conduct were devised, published and circulated to hospitals, nursing homes and to members of the medical profession.[16]

By 1896, Agnes Hunt and Emily Goodford were living and working in Ollerton. The Society of Trained Masseuses was thriving and, at its first Annual General Meeting, it was decided to invite patronage from a number of respected medical practitioners supportive of the society and its objectives. With a membership of 250 in 1900 the society changed its name to the Incorporated Society of Trained Masseuses (ISTMS) acquiring the legal and public status of a professional organisation.[17]

Mrs Hunt, Agnes's mother, had stayed in London following the family's return to England from Australia, working energetically for the Charity Organisation Society. During the eleven years she had lived in the capital, she had seen all her children reach adulthood and all but Agnes marry. Tragically, two of her daughters had died during this period, one in childbirth, the other from diabetes.[18] On hearing of the terminal illness of one of her sons from pulmonary tuberculosis, she determined to make the long journey to his San Francisco home to pay a final extended visit to his family. Mrs Hunt travelled to America in 1898 and, in the following year, was joined by Agnes who also wished to spend some time with her dying brother and his family.

When Mrs Hunt decided her visit should come to an end, Agnes left to accompany her mother on the long journey home. During the return journey to England, Mrs Hunt announced to her startled daughter that, as she was now too old and too deaf to continue with her work in London, she was in future going to live with Agnes. She had obviously been considering her future for some time and had decided that Agnes, a trained and experienced nurse in addition to being her only unmarried daughter, was the most appropriate person to care for her during her declining years. Agnes caught a brief glimpse of a bleak future as companion/nurse to her aging mother, but before she had fully comprehended the full effect her mother's decision would have on her life and chosen career, Mrs Hunt offered an alternative. She said she had heard that Florence House was empty and was available for rent. This property was part of the family estates in Baschurch, Shropshire, where Agnes had spent her childhood years while living at the nearby Boreatton Hall.

Florence House was suitable, in Mrs Hunt's opinion, for use as a convalescent home for the Salop Infirmary, and she announced she would give Agnes £200 a year to pay rent, taxes and the cook's wages. In addition, she would pay half the gardener's wages and also pay an agreed rate for hospitality for visitors who would come to stay at the house.[19]

Agnes had many reservations about her mother's idea and, on her return to Ollerton, discussed the proposal with Emily, who was equally concerned, particularly about the overall funding of the proposed venture. By pooling their limited resources, Emily calculated they would have £500, a very small amount with which to run a convalescent home. Agnes's main reservations focused on the Salop Infirmary's wishes regarding the establishment of a convalescent home, the compliance or otherwise of the medical and surgical staff, and the suitability of the selected venue with regard to the water supply and drainage.

Despite their concerns, Agnes Hunt and Emily Goodford resigned from their posts, packed their belongings and left Ollerton for Baschurch. On arrival, they discovered the euphoria of Mrs Hunt's description of Florence House was far from the reality they faced. The house was dusty, dirty and malodorous, having been empty for at least six years before their arrival, and was surrounded by a totally overgrown, unkempt garden. Neither the drains nor the water supply were in an acceptable condition and, although the proposal for a convalescent home had been met with enthusiasm by medical and surgical staff in the area, the management team of the Salop Infirmary was not at all enthusiastic. Emily Goodford summarised the despair they felt on their arrival in Baschurch by commenting with bitterness and asperity that it was unfortunate that Agnes's mother had not remained in America.[20]

Having made preliminary decisions about apportionment of space, and having identified and temporarily resolved most of the problems with the water supply and sewage disposal, they established a committee to run the proposed convalescent home. Key figures on this committee were Eliza Kenyon as honorary treasurer who, with meticulous care and ability, steered the home through its early years of uncertain funding and Florence Marianne Hunt, who was the appointed joint secretary with Miss Polly Lloyd. Archdeacon Maude was nominated Chairman and the local vicar also served on the committee and acted as chaplain to the home.

With its administrative support structure in place and the rooms clean though sparsely furnished, the Baschurch Convalescent Home opened its doors to the first patients on 1 October 1900. The prime instigator for the establishment of the convalescent home at Baschurch had been Florence Marianne Hunt, Agnes' mother. She acted as honorary secretary during its early years, generously supporting the home through its many financial difficulties. Having previously worked as a charity fundraiser in London for a number of years she brought her skills and experience to the wholehearted support of the home, pursuing friends and relatives with ruthless determination and intense zeal. Early in March 1914, at the age of seventy-seven, Mrs Hunt suffered a left-sided stroke which paralysed her right arm and leg. She was not an easy patient to nurse and, although she regained use in her arm, she was never to walk again. In October 1917, she died following a fall sustained some five months previously.[21]

NOTES

[1] Hunt, Dame Agnes, *This is My Life*, London, Blackie, 1938

[2] *The Heritage of Oswestry – The origin and development of the Robert Jones and Agnes Hunt Orthopaedic Hospital, Oswestry, 1900–1975,* Oswestry, The Robert Jones and Agnes Hunt Orthopaedic Hospital, 1975

[3] Hunt, *This is My Life*, op. cit.

[4] Ibid

[5] *The Heritage of Oswestry,* 1975, op. cit.

[6] Hunt, *This is My Life*, op. cit.

[7] Ibid

[8] Ibid

[9] Ibid

[10] Carter, M., *Healing & Hope*, Robert Jones and Agnes Hunt Orthopaedic and District NHS Trust, 2000

[11] Hunt, *This is My Life*, op. cit.

[12] Ibid

[13] Wicksteed, J., *The Growth of a Profession*, London, Edward Arnold, 1948

[14] Young, P., 'A Short History of the Chartered Society of Physiotherapy', *Physiotherapy*, vol 55 no 7 pp 271–278, 1969

[15] Ibid

[16] Tidswell, M.E., 'Physiotherapy: A True Profession?', unpublished MA dissertation, 1991

[17] Young, P., 'A Short History of the Chartered Society of Physiotherapy', op. cit.

[18] Hunt, *This is My Life*, op. cit.

[19] Ibid

[20] Ibid

[21] Carter, M., *Healing & Hope*, Robert Jones and Agnes Hunt Orthopaedic and District NHS Trust, 2000

Chapter 3
Baschurch Convalescent Home: 1900–1909

By October 1900, Agnes was in her early thirties and had been crippled for more than twenty years. Despite having endured considerable pain and significant disability, she had led an active life, and had trained and worked as a nurse in physically arduous conditions. It was during her training and subsequent nursing career that she had developed ideas she would now put into practice. Many of her nursing experiences had involved the treatment of cripples from disadvantaged backgrounds and it was the contrast between the conditions suffered by these crippled children raised in poverty and her own experiences of a sheltered, protective environment with the security of an assured income that made her want to help others with disabling conditions. This was reinforced by her later experiences in nursing and confirmed her desire to help fellow cripples throughout her life.[1] She was now prepared and ready to embark on a venture that was destined to revolutionise treatment for people with chronic disabling conditions and to alter public attitudes towards them.

From her first days of nursing at Rhyl, she had learned that fresh air and a healthy diet were essential components of any successful treatment for cripples and this she incorporated into the ethos of care at Baschurch. Also following her traumatic experiences as a lady pupil nurse at the West London Hospital, she had vowed that if she ever rose to the rank of matron, no young person she employed to care for the sick would suffer any deterioration in her health as a direct result of the work. Although the work at Baschurch was always very hard, the living conditions and the nourishment of patients and staff alike ensured they remained healthy.

Once the Baschurch Convalescent Home came into being, it became very popular with and was used extensively by surgeons and physicians practising in the area. The regime of care developed by the home was uncomplicated but effective. Plenty of rest, good food and fresh air were the key factors in a programme that followed the pattern of treatment Agnes had experienced in her own home as a child following the onset of her hip problems. The final ingredient of the care package was happiness. Its inclusion was the result of her childhood experiences and had been reinforced during her time as a lady pupil at the Royal Alexandra Hospital, Rhyl, where she had started her nurse training. Agnes Hunt and Emily Goodford, the nominated joint superintendents of the convalescent home, were inundated by the numbers of children referred for periods of convalescence or to build up their strength and confidence prior to surgery.[2] The sick and crippled children admitted gained strength from the home's care package and were then enabled to withstand and even overcome many of the diseases that threatened to overwhelm them and for which there was as yet no effective medication.

Prior to the opening, two first-floor rooms had been designated for use as wards for the care of the children admitted for treatment. However, once the home became operational, it was obvious that as the only means of access to these rooms was by a very steep staircase, it was too dangerous for staff to consider carrying the children from one floor to the other. As there was only five pounds in the home's reserve fund, it was agreed it was not practical to consider moving the staircase, altering its slope or undertaking any major structural alteration to the rented property. The only solution was to restrict the use of the accommodation on the first floor to children who were relatively independent, able to walk with or without some assistance and who were considered to be safe when climbing the staircase.[3]

This situation was of considerable concern to the joint superintendents as it now appeared that the children who would benefit most from the home's innovative approach to their disabling conditions would be denied access to the facility because of the physical nature of the building. Not a person to be discouraged by difficult problems, Agnes pondered, made a few inquiries and devised an ingenious solution. Some disused empty sheds were 'borrowed' from Boreatton Park, now the family home of Agnes's eldest brother, Rowland, who was in South Africa fighting in the Boer War. The sheds were dismantled, transported to Florence House and re-erected in the garden. The home's tiny reserve fund was used to provide a concrete floor for the structure and, in 1901, the first of the now famous open-sided wards came into being. This ensured that children who were too crippled to cope with the stairs leading to the designated wards on the first floor were able to receive and benefit from the special care offered by the home as originally planned.[4] The following year, twenty-five pounds was raised to build another open-sided ward to expand the number of young patients who could be accepted for the effective open air treatment.[5] Children treated by this revolutionary regime of fresh air and good food appeared to thrive with no sign of coughs, colds or other minor ailments. Relatives, however, were on occasion less enthusiastic about the spartan conditions and one mother, who rejected the treatment offered by the home, is reported as saying she would prefer to follow her child to the grave rather than allow it to sleep in an open shed.[6]

Agnes had a further recurrence of her hip problem during 1903 and on this occasion was advised to consult Robert Jones, a forward-thinking surgeon with a robust sense of humour and a practice based at the Southern Hospital Liverpool.[7] The second half of the nineteenth century had been a time of rapid development of surgery. As procedures were refined, the skills of practitioners increased and surgical specialisms were developed, including orthopaedics, in which Robert Jones was a leading exponent. Robert Jones had training in 'modern' surgery, using anaesthesia and antisepsis to support his work. He was very progressive in his ideas, striving to advance orthopaedic surgical techniques. A great humanitarian, he spent much of his time with the underprivileged children around the Liverpool dockland and slum areas.[8] He was interested particularly in improving the physical capabilities of the numerous children in his practice who were crippled by disease, under-nutrition or deformity. Robert Jones was, by the turn of the twentieth century, able to offer crippled children hope of a considerably improved quality of life. This came from his enlightened approach to the management of their physical problems and the introduction of aseptic procedures in hospitals combined with improved nursing practices that reduced post-operative morbidity and mortality.

At some time during her prolonged course of treatment, Agnes invited Robert Jones to visit the Baschurch Convalescent Home to observe her work with crippled children. It appeared to her that they had similar ideals and were, in their different approaches, enabling crippled children to develop more of their potential, giving them hope for the future and contributing to general improvement in their prospects. Robert Jones was impressed by his visit to Baschurch where the continuity of treatment for crippled children he had so long advocated was being carried out routinely. He had experienced many frustrations resulting from the habitual early discharge of his patients from hospital before they experienced the full benefit of surgery, and he expressed his unqualified approval of the care being given to the young patients at Baschurch. He was very enthusiastic about the treatment regimes she had developed and offered Agnes the opportunity to take the children in her care for outpatient appointments to his Liverpool consulting rooms.

The first patients from Baschurch to benefit from this arrangement were seen as outpatients in Liverpool during December 1903[9] and, four months later, Robert Jones accepted the invitation to be honorary consulting surgeon to the home.[10] He was pleased to support an institution whose ideals matched his own endeavours and, from the outset of this association, invited surgeons from many different countries to visit the facility to observe the pioneering open air treatment of TB and other diseases[11] before they returned to their native shores to practise the additional skills they had learned on their visit to England. The Baschurch Convalescent Home impressed the visitors as it was believed to be the only institution in the country at the time to treat patients with hip disease and TB affectations entirely in the open air.[12] These overseas consultants were generally very positive in their comments, considering Baschurch to be the best facility they had seen, as it consistently produced excellent results against a background of a very low individual cost.[13]

Robert Jones's acceptance of the honorary consulting

surgeon's post changed the status of the home from that of purely a convalescent home to an institution where surgical cases were treated routinely and where, it could be anticipated, operations would be performed from time to time.[14] Hospital status had been granted and it was agreed that Mr Jones would visit Baschurch each month in order to fulfil his obligations to the young patients. With this arrangement in place, the children would be saved the long but exciting journey to Liverpool for consultation and Robert Jones would be in a position to operate on the most needy children on his regular visits to Shropshire.

Agnes and Emily were delighted by the rapid development of their project and, despite the lack of an operating theatre, they were not daunted by the thought of providing appropriate facilities. Both had gained a thorough training and had experience in antiseptic methods. They accepted that, if surgery was to be undertaken at Baschurch, a room had to be provided in which Robert Jones could undertake surgical procedures and operate under aseptic conditions.[15] Prior to each visit by the surgeon, the room chosen for use as a temporary operating theatre was totally stripped, then scrubbed throughout with carbolic solution. Towels, bowls and surgical instruments were boiled in fish kettles and other large receptacles to sterilise them thoroughly and, on the first visit, after lighting failed, the first operating session was finally drawn to a successful conclusion using two candles to provide the necessary lighting in the room that was normally used as the dining room.[16]

The absence of a separate dedicated operating theatre was obviously an inconvenience and eventually, in 1907, one was built, equipped and furnished.[17] There was also a surgeons' dressing room, a sterilising room and a large annex which was used as post-operative recovery space on operating weekends and as a children's playroom the rest of the time.[18]

The home was significantly under-financed from the outset and had survived the early years only as a result of the many financial self-sacrifices made by Agnes and by the generosity of family and friends who provided much-needed clothing, beds, bedding and equipment required to support the nursing care of the patients.[19] Agnes received no salary in 1904 as the account for the home was overdrawn. Also, over the next three years, she paid the wages for an extra nurse, the housekeeper and a parlour maid. The porters, who also made splints for the patients, were paid by Agnes, who also provided and nurtured the pony used to carry the children on outings and picnics around the area.[20]

Patients were obviously unaware of the major financial problems of the hospital and it continued to act as a magnet to crippled children, overwhelming the small staff with the numbers of needy people seeking assistance. Adult women had been admitted for treatment from 1905[21] and this increased significantly the level of nursing care that had to be provided.

During 1906, a concentrated fundraising effort resulted in Agnes being reimbursed most of her previous excess expenditure. At the same time, operational procedures were reviewed and as a result, financial responsibility for the day-to-day organisation of the hospital transferred from Agnes and Emily to a committee that established the enterprise on a more businesslike basis. In theory, this gave the joint superintendents more time to concentrate on issues relating to the practical nursing care of the patients admitted to the hospital.

Despite this financial realignment, Agnes continued to buy necessary pieces of equipment for the hospital when required, due to insufficient financial resources supporting the enterprise. One such purchase was the steriliser she bought for use in the operating theatre in 1906.[22]

By 1908, the patient profile of the hospital had altered radically from that of the convalescent home at its opening in 1900. Patients suffering pulmonary tuberculosis had been transferred to sanatoria and convalescent patients were no longer accommodated in the hospital. Women with orthopaedic problems now occupied the beds vacated by these patient groups. These new patients required more nursing care than the children they replaced and they were also much slower to mobilise once their period of bed rest was completed. More fully trained and qualified nurses were required to cope with the new challenges presented. To satisfy this requirement, Agnes and Emily had to determine a strategy that had a possibility of success and would allow the hospital to continue its valuable work. Money, as always, was in very short supply and, as Agnes could not afford to pay for any further additional nurses from her own personal resources, an alternative solution had to be found.

After much discussion, Agnes and Emily decided to offer training in orthopaedic nursing to suitable young ladies. This of necessity had to be a course for pupil nurses who would not only provide their own uniforms but who also would expect no salary. If the course were to be offered to student nurses, the hospital would have to provide uniforms and also recompense participants with a small training allowance. This was not a financial option at this particular time. On completion of a one-year specialist course in orthopaedic nursing, the proposal was that the pupil nurses would transfer to a general hospital to complete registered nurse training.[23]

The proposal had considerable merit but, in fact, did little to solve the major staffing problems that beset the hospital. Pupil nurses proved to be reluctant to leave at the end of the year to continue with their training in general nursing. A certificate awarded to successful candidates on completion of the course, demonstrating that training had been undertaken in orthopaedic nursing, had no validity outside the hospital and was considered to be unmarketable. The superintendents continued to be significantly overworked and accepted there was little prospect of their continuing the level of activity required to operate the hospital with its existing patient load and small staff. The point was about to be reached when they would no longer be able to cater for the needs of adult patients who were less resilient to hardship than the children.

Agnes had spent many long hours over several months considering the situation in which they now found themselves without reaching an acceptable solution to their overwhelming problems. She had considered all possible options including borrowing money to enable the hospital to continue in its present form. Finally, one warm, slightly overcast day in May 1909, she had the idea for which she had been searching all these months. The germ of a plan that could secure the long-term survival of the hospital and prove to be her salvation. She hurried, as much as she was able, to find her friend, Emily, with whom she discussed everything before taking any action.

Developments in health care often occur during periods of war or following major social upheaval. During the late eighteenth and early nineteenth centuries, there had been significant displacement of country people towards areas where new industries had been established. This effectively destroyed the centuries-old population balance of the country. Urban migration produced intense overcrowding in the rapidly developing cities with attendant problems of poor sanitation and inadequate supplies of pure drinking water. Slums were created where disease was rife, infant mortality high, despair and violence the norm and grinding poverty reigned supreme. Under-nutrition, intense drudgery and a continual struggle for existence was all that many of the population could hope for.

When she first opened the convalescent home, Agnes Hunt recruited her child patients from the slum areas of Liverpool and rural Shropshire and, by 1909, she had clearly demonstrated to the world the therapeutic value of rest, good food and fresh air for the successful care of cripples. Many of her young patients first experienced a nutritious balanced diet, appropriate to the needs of their developing bodies, on admission to the Baschurch Convalescent Home. Agnes was reluctant to reduce the level of her activities as she felt it would be a betrayal of the patients she had pledged to serve.

In several areas of the country, small groups of nurses who were also trained in massage and medical rubbing techniques were forming associations, institutes or guilds. These highly trained nurses had, by their efforts, been successful in identifying massage as a therapeutic modality, distancing it from the unsavoury image from which it had previously suffered, so that it was by 1909 accepted by the medical profession as a valid treatment technique. The most successful of these organisations was the Incorporated Society of Trained Masseuses (ISTMS), started by nurses from the London Hospital in 1894, but there were others – for example, the Northern Guild based in Manchester and the Faculty of Physiotherapy based in Glasgow.

In her search for improved staffing levels and the continued enhancement of the standard of care being given to her patients, Agnes had already heard of these new approaches to treatment and considered many of her patients would benefit from the application of massage before they were allowed out of bed after many months of recumbency.[24] She had considered carefully the particular problems associated with rehabilitation of adult patients and had observed they were slower than the children to mobilise after completion of their prescribed periods of bed rest. She had heard also that the ISTMS offered courses and examinations in massage and medical rubbing, and decided to investigate further.

With Emily's encouragement, Agnes made inquiries about the possibility of training her nurses in the skills of massage and, in 1909, requested the hospital be recognised as a training school for this purpose. A year later, in 1910, the ISTMS offered an additional course and examination in Swedish remedial exercise to candidates who already held a certificate of Competency in Massage,[25] and this was added to the hospital's repertoire. These diverse options provided the answer to many of the hospital's staffing problems.

Pupil nurses were now able to undertake a course in orthopaedic nursing followed by another in massage and Swedish remedial exercise. The programmes of study would be devised and implemented by the hospital in which they worked and, on successful completion of the ISTMS examinations, candidates would be awarded the society's certificate. This would enable those pupil nurses who did not want to leave Baschurch at the end of the year to complete a further course of training to gain a recognised qualification supported by a marketable certificate.[26] It also helped to solve the most pressing staffing needs of the hospital at little extra cost. Patients benefited from the diversification of treatment by the addition of massage and Swedish remedial exercise, and a new era in the life of the hospital was about to start.

NOTES

[1] Hunt, Dame Agnes, *This is My Life*, London, Blackie, 1938

[2] Carter, M., *Healing & Hope*, Robert Jones and Agnes Hunt Orthopaedic and District NHS Trust, 2000

[3] Extracts from the report of the meeting of the Annual Subscribers of the Baschurch Convalescent Home, 15 October 1903

[4] Hunt, Dame Agnes, *This is My Life*, op. cit.

[5] Hunt, Dame Agnes, *This is My Life*, London, Blackie, 1938

[6] Extracts from the minutes of the General Committee of the Baschurch Convalescent Home, 14 September 1903

[7] Hunt, *This is My Life*, op. cit.

[8] *The Heritage of Oswestry – The origin and development of the Robert Jones and Agnes Hunt Orthopaedic Hospital, Oswestry, 1900–1975,* Oswestry, The Robert Jones and Agnes Hunt Orthopaedic Hospital, 1975

[9] Hunt, *This is My Life*, op. cit.

[10] Ibid

[11] Extracts from the minutes of the Annual General Meeting of the Baschurch Convalescent Home, 13 October 1904

[12] Extracts from the minutes of the Executive Committee meeting of the Baschurch Convalescent Home, 25 July 1908

[13] Extracts from the minutes of the Executive Committee meeting of Baschurch Convalescent Home, 27 October 1906

[14] Extracts from the minutes of the Executive Committee meeting of Baschurch Convalescent Home, 17 July 1905

[15] Hunt, *This is My Life*, op. cit.

[16] Ibid

[17] Extracts from the minutes of the quarterly meeting of the Baschurch Convalescent Home, 14 September 1907

[18] Carter, M., *Healing & Hope*, Robert Jones and Agnes Hunt Orthopaedic and District NHS Trust, 2000

[19] Extracts from the minutes of the Annual General Meeting of the Baschurch Convalescent Home, 13 October 1904

[20] Extracts from the minutes of the General Committee of the Baschurch Convalescent Home, 11 April 1905

[21] Carter, M., *Healing & Hope*, op. cit.

[22] Extracts from the Annual Report of the Baschurch Convalescent Home, 1906–1907

[23] Hunt, *This is My Life*, op. cit.

[24] Ibid

[25] Chartered Society of Physiotherapy, '100 years 1894–1994', *Physiotherapy* vol. 80 issue A, 1994

[26] Carter, M., *Healing & Hope*, Robert Jones and Agnes Hunt Orthopaedic and District NHS Trust, 2000

Chapter 4
Early Years of the School of Massage: 1909–1920

From its tentative start as a convalescent home for crippled children, Baschurch had expanded and developed into a hospital overflowing with crippled men, women and children from the slums of Liverpool, Shropshire and the Potteries. Here, Agnes Hunt and Emily Goodford, with superb orthopaedic skill, nursed and straightened twisted limbs, set children on their feet and taught them skills for the future.[1] Over the years the hospital had been in operation, Agnes had observed that, whereas children normally mobilised without assistance once splints and restraints were removed, adults required more skilled nursing care during the resting phase of their treatment. They were also apprehensive and lacking in confidence once the splints were removed and were very slow to start moving about normally. They needed constant encouragement and assistance to return to their normal levels of activity.

By 1909, more qualified staff were needed to care effectively for the increased numbers of patients treated and to share the personal and professional burden of management of the hospital shouldered by Agnes and assisted by Emily. As the hospital was privately owned and funded mainly by the generosity of family and a network of 'Friends', it was always under extreme financial pressure and, to ensure its continued existence, the joint superintendents were required to conduct all aspects of the hospital's activities and development at minimal cost.

The proposal to extend the orthopaedic nursing training developed at Baschurch to include a course in massage and medical rubbing had every chance of success as it was devised to be implemented from within current staff resources and so would not incur additional cost to the hospital. In 1910, a further course in Swedish remedial exercise became available for people already qualified from the course in massage. This extended the curriculum and effectively consolidated the learning opportunities without increasing financial responsibilities for the course organisers.[2]

It also provided a limited income generation capability as it was decided by Agnes and Emily that tuition, already in place for those students who had trained as orthopaedic nurses, could be extended to accommodate additional candidates who wished to take the courses in massage and Swedish remedial exercise alone. In this situation, a fee of one pound per week was to be charged for course tuition.[3]

In comparison with the number and complexity of the procedures required nowadays before an undergraduate course in physiotherapy can be established, the new School of Massage at Baschurch was started with incredible ease. At that time, provided an acceptable curriculum of study had been submitted to, and accepted by, the ISTMS Council and two testimonials had been received from medical practitioners, the institution could enter candidates aged twenty-one years or more to the examinations of the Incorporated Society of Trained Masseuses.[4]

Students who preferred to remain at Baschurch once they had finished training in orthopaedic nursing could now continue their studies at the hospital to gain a nationally recognised professional qualification on successful completion of the ISTMS courses and examinations. They were then available for employment by the hospital, or elsewhere, as trained staff.

Patients, particularly the adults, gained immediate benefit from the increased range of treatments available at the hospital, and approximately twenty daily massage programmes were implemented as part of the training course. This did not go unnoticed by Robert Jones, who immediately recognised the therapeutic value of massage for his patients and complimented Agnes and her staff for being so forward-looking as to incorporate this 'new' regime of treatment into the hospital's care package. It was of obvious benefit to patients, aiding their return to normal functional activity levels more effectively than had previously been the case.[5]

The professional viability of the hospital had never been

doubted, but its basis of funding, the level of equipment provision and low staffing levels meant it was always in a precarious position. By developing the combined course in orthopaedic nursing, massage and remedial exercise, Agnes eased the staffing position for probationers and created opportunity for the recruitment of qualified staff. Indeed, during the first few years of the course's operation, five qualifiers remained at the hospital, appointed as ward sisters and masseuses.[6]

The programme proved popular, with the majority of candidates taking the combined course to complete professional registration. Three students, Dorothy Hayden, Dorothy Wood and Jane Field, enrolled on the first course and were trained by a Miss F. Porter. Two of the candidates qualified at the first attempt, but the third, Jane Field, failed practical massage and successfully retook the examination in February 1912.[7] Of the first group to qualify from Baschurch, Dorothy Wood is thought to have started a school of massage and medical gymnastics at Manchester Royal Infirmary in 1919 as she trained and submitted a candidate for the profession's examinations in 1921. Another, Dorothy Hayden, was related to a later course qualifier, Decima Hayden, superintendent physiotherapist at the hospital during the 1950s. The first three courses provided a total of nine qualified masseuses trained in orthopaedic nursing for the profession, enabling dissemination of their highly developed expertise across the country.

Although the training facility appeared to be running effectively, detailed arrangements of course implementation were not observed directly by representatives from the Incorporated Society of Trained Masseuses until the course had been in operation for five years. History does not record the allocation of time on this first visit during 1915, but one can imagine Florence Marianne Hunt played a key role holding court over afternoon tea taken in her sitting room, while regaling the visitors with her version of the efficacy of the new training courses. Irrespective of the details of the programme arranged, the report received following this visit and inspection of the school's organisation proved satisfactory and approval was given for the training methods used and for the general management of the courses offered.[8]

Owing to the pressure on space, treatments were given only to ward-based bedridden patients and, after some time, staff complained of the restrictions imposed by this arrangement. The hospital had appointed a qualified Swedish remedial gymnast/masseuse in 1914 who explained that full use of her specific expertise required more space than was available in a ward and a firmer base for individual treatments than that provided by a bed. On fine days, exercises could be given in the open air, but this was not an option when the weather was inclement. These issues were raised and coincided with a proposal to acquire some of the estate buildings attached to Boreatton Hall, the estate that had been in the Hunt family for centuries and in which Agnes had spent her unconventional childhood. The purchase of these buildings gave the hospital room for expansion to relieve the intense pressure on existing facilities at Florence House. There were at the time about sixty-five patients receiving daily massage and/or electrical treatments.[9] The purchase was to provide a long shed to ease the overcrowding of the Baschurch site[10] and provide space for a dedicated massage room large enough to accommodate the teaching of Swedish remedial exercises.[11] As with most of the hospital's facilities, the room was to be used for other activities and was not destined to be used exclusively for treatment purposes.

Following the outbreak of the First World War in Europe, Florence Marianne Hunt offered approximately a hundred beds at Baschurch for the care of wounded soldiers and attention was immediately directed to the emergency practical training of Voluntary Aid Detachment (VAD) nurses to cope with the expected trauma cases. From October that year until the end of the war, wounded soldiers occupied the wards previously used for the treatment of women. The orthopaedic patients displaced to provide trauma beds at the hospital were accommodated in the facilities that had been created at Boreatton Hall.

With the addition of wounded and convalescent soldiers to the complement of patients in the hospital, there was a pressing need for additional probationer nurses to provide an acceptable level of care. Most of the probationer nurses who became students training during the First World War were VAD nurses recruited from county families. Before they started attending to the needs of the wounded soldiers, Dame Agnes advised the nurses not to become too friendly with them. She identified that the patients were mainly of the same social class as gardeners employed by the probationers' families although they were now in uniform and fighting for their country.[12]

It was difficult to find rooms for these extra nurses as any accommodation that became available was soon filled and they slept in a variety of temporary accommodations which included horse boxes, wooden huts, caravans, draughty attics, in rented accommodation in Baschurch village and in the servants' quarters at Boreatton Hall. For Agnes Hunt, the most important thing was the effective and efficient care of the patients. She rejected the hierarchical relationships she had met in the large hospitals in London and treated all her staff with equal respect. From the first day on the wards, nurses, up to and including Agnes herself, were called 'Sister'. This did not please those nurses who were fully trained and qualified, but it was the tradition at Baschurch. Students wore blue fitted overalls and caps and as the wards were open-sided, often wore several layers of additional clothing underneath the overalls to combat the cold. Despite the lack of heating and the open air work, both patients and staff were very healthy.[13]

Pressure from doctors and masseuses working in military hospitals had encouraged the ISTMS Council to establish a curriculum in medical electricity so that electrical modalities could be used to treat the trauma cases.[14] Gunshot wounds and fractured limbs were now a regular feature in the hospital and Agnes considered she might be obliged to recruit and pay a salary to a person capable of implementing these new treatments instead of relying on the massage and exercise of the existing training programme. Student training in the new techniques would also have to be considered, probably following the established pattern of training used by the hospital for the training in massage.

From the establishment of the school, massage training had been provided to successful orthopaedic nursing candidates, without cost, provided they accepted an unsalaried service commitment to the nursing of patients for the duration of their studies.[15] The programme was implemented successfully and the practice of offering free tuition in physiotherapy to nurses who had trained at the hospital continued until the combined orthopaedic nursing/physiotherapy courses ceased in the late 1960s.

Later, in the mid 1980s, there was an attempt made to identify realistic tuition fees for courses in physiotherapy and the annual tuition fee for the course offered by the Oswestry-based school was set by hospital management at twenty pounds per year or sixty pounds per course. This fee was six pounds less than the original charge determined by Agnes Hunt as appropriate for the first six-month course of instruction in massage and Swedish remedial exercise in 1909 and was totally unrealistic seventy years later. The battle for a more appropriate course tuition fee was hard won at local level finally to bring the school in line with other national institutions offering physiotherapy courses with a tuition fee set initially at £1,000 per annum.

Tuition and preparation for the ISTMS examinations continued during the war with students studying for their examinations in addition to fulfilling their ward duties. Anatomy classes were held in an unheated room over a butcher's shop in Baschurch from 05.00–07.30 each morning and students also learned about electrical treatments and nerve testing in addition to massage and remedial exercises. Examinations were taken at a centre in Liverpool, and Baschurch students, despite the difficulties they had experienced in finding adequate study time due to their nursing duties, had a high level of success throughout the war years.[16]

Once the war was over and relative normality was restored to the hospital, Miss E.C. Pearce, a certificated teacher of massage and medical gymnastics, was appointed in 1920 to complete the training of both probationer nurses and massage students. Later, in 1927, after she had left Shropshire to work elsewhere, she wrote the first definitive text on orthopaedic nursing.

Miss Pearce's appointment heralded recognition of some of the deficits of the training offered by the hospital. It had been penalised by its success and training courses had been established primarily to induce a steady supply of willing helpers to cope with the increasing nursing needs of the patients. No thought had been given initially to the academic needs of these pupils, but with Miss Pearce's appointment, steps were taken to remedy the situation with consideration of the allocation of defined study time and increased teaching input. The benefits of this improved organisation were obvious immediately as three pupils entered the ISTMS examinations in 1920 and, by the following year, thirteen students were prepared for entry.[17]

At this time, the ISTMS organised separate courses for the physiotherapy components with examinations and certificates awarded for proven competence in massage, remedial exercise and medical electricity. The format of examination that had been established was for viva voce, practical and written papers in each of the three areas with additional testing of anatomical knowledge and physiological understanding. The examination results quoted for the school for 1921, and for which Miss Pearce was justifiably congratulated, reflect the multiplicity of these hurdles for candidates and teachers alike. During the year, six candidates entered and obtained the certificate in remedial gymnastics and one entered and obtained the certificate in massage. In addition, one candidate entered and passed part one of the remedial gymnastics examination and another entered and passed part one of the combined massage and remedial gymnastics examination.[18]

The hospital did not have the facilities to train students for examinations in medical electricity although it is recorded that patients were receiving this form of treatment as early as 1915. History does not record, however, who was actually treating the patients with this new modality. It was a time of relative freedom; professions were not as regulated as they are now and inter-professional boundaries were blurred. Neither patients nor staff had even minimum regulation or protection. Fortunately in most instances, treatment programmes were completed without problems being encountered. It is, however, a little daunting to discover that, as late as 1931,[19] when the hospital's qualified radiographer became ill and was on extended sick leave, the matron's secretary undertook his duties in addition to her own secretarial work.

During 1920 the Incorporated Society of Trained Masseuses

merged with the Manchester-based Institute of Massage and Remedial Gymnastics. It was in this year also that the society was granted a Royal Charter confirming its position as the leading organisation in the country for the training of massage and medical gymnastics. The name of the professional organisation was changed to the Chartered Society of Massage and Medical Gymnastics (CSMMG), a name it carried until 1943.[20] A new system of testing students' competence to practise, the Conjoint Examination, was devised and implemented nationally in 1922. This should not be confused with the examinations of the same name organised by Agnes Hunt to test competencies in orthopaedic nursing and massage. The term has been used in this text exclusively to identify the national examinations of the Chartered Society of Massage and Medical Gymnastics.

The facilities at Baschurch had been significantly overstretched for many years with water supplies and drainage systems constantly causing great concern. It is a tribute to the level of hygiene practised at the hospital that there was, during these early years, no serious outbreak of waterborne diseases such as diphtheria or typhoid fever. The premises were totally inadequate for the level and volume of work undertaken. Patients were accommodated in assorted converted farm buildings and a series of ramshackle open-sided sheds scattered over several acres of land, but their living conditions were very much better than those endured by the superintendents and staff. For example, a disused pigsty was converted first for use as a plaster room and then became a sitting room in which Agnes and Emily were able to spend their few short hours of relaxation. At that stage, a new plaster room was created by conversion of the coach house. A small dairy building was used as bathroom, store room and bicycle store, two long cowsheds were converted to wards for the accommodation of twenty to twenty-six patients in each and there were several open-sided sheds each accommodating sixteen to eighteen beds.[21]

Probationer nurses lived in converted horseboxes which were notoriously cold in winter.[22] They wore warm skirts and jerseys underneath their uniform issue white cotton overalls as they spent most of their time caring for patients in the open-sided sheds, walking from one of the scattered buildings to another almost always without shade or protection from the vagaries of the English weather.[23] Although patients were always well nourished, when money was short, staff were the first to suffer.[24] Their diet was boring, lacked nutrition and, in many instances, was of insufficient quantity and quality to provide the energy required for the arduous duties they were required to perform. Working hours were long, often with only a few hours' respite during the afternoons, but, despite the hardship they endured, Nurses' memories of their time at Baschurch stress the happiness and inspiration they gained from working under the leadership provided by Agnes Hunt and Emily Goodford.[25]

Finally, the war ended and, once the last of the military patients were discharged in 1919, an expert inspected the drains at Baschurch and condemned them as a public health risk. Sanitation and drainage had been a problem for the home since it first opened and now it was imperative that new premises were found to avert closure of the hospital.[26] As a result of the extensive search undertaken over several counties, the site of the Park Hall Military Hospital at Gobowen was identified in 1919. This was a popular choice as it was only a few miles north of Baschurch and could be altered with very little cost to make an open-air hospital to accommodate 320 patients.[27]

The buildings at Park Hall were in poor shape having been erected for temporary use for the duration of the war and now, in 1919, many of them were ready for replacement by permanent structures or for demolition. With significant financial grants from the Red Cross and Shropshire War Memorial Societies, the site was purchased and, after many months of hard work, by 1 February 1921, patients were transferred to their new home, now named the Shropshire Orthopaedic Hospital. This marked the definitive closure of Florence House and the Baschurch Home passed into memory.[28]

After a friendship and working partnership with Agnes Hunt spanning thirty years, Emily Goodford, co-founder and co-honorary superintendent of the Baschurch Home, died after a short illness in 1920. This was a devastating blow to Agnes who, having already lost her mother and several of her siblings, was now without the companionship and wise counsel of her longtime friend. Emily never saw the patients transferred to the new hospital site at Park Hall[29] but her name lives on, initially in the naming of the hospital chapel and then as a ward on the main corridor of the hospital. This ward was converted for use as the Day Case Surgery Unit in the late 1990s.

NOTES

[1] Taylor, F.M., unpublished staff memories of Baschurch, 1914–1917

[2] Chartered Society of Physiotherapy, '100 years 1894–1994', *Physiotherapy* vol. 80 issue A, 1994

[3] Extracts from the Annual Report of the Baschurch Convalescent Home, 1912

[4] Chartered Society of Physiotherapy, '100 years 1894–1994', op. cit.

[5] Extracts from the minutes of the Annual General Meeting of the Baschurch Convalescent Home, 30 September 1911

[6] Extracts from the Annual Report of the Baschurch Home, 1914–1915

[7] Extracts from the minutes of the Council of the Incorporated Society of Trained Masseuses

[8] Extracts from the Annual Report of the Baschurch Home, 1915–1916

[9] Extracts from the Minutes of the Executive Committee Meeting of the Baschurch Home, September 1915

[10] Hunt, Dame Agnes, *This is My Life*, London, Blackie, 1938

[11] Extracts from the Minutes of the Executive Committee Meeting of the Baschurch Home, 12 March 1914

[12] Lovatt, P., unpublished student memories, 1916–1919

[13] Taylor, F., unpublished staff memories of Baschurch, 1914–1917

[14] Chartered Society of Physiotherapy, '100 years 1894–1994', op. cit.

[15] Extracts from the minutes of the Executive Committee meeting of the Baschurch Home, December 1916

[16] Taylor, F., student memories, op. cit.

[17] Extracts from the Annual Report of the Baschurch Home, 1920

[18] Extracts from the Annual Report of the Shropshire Orthopaedic Hospital, 1921

[19] Extracts from the minutes of the House Committee meeting of the Shropshire Orthopaedic Hospital, 15 June 1931

[20] Chartered Society of Physiotherapy, '100 years 1894–1994', *Physiotherapy* vol. 80 issue A, 1994

[21] Abrahams, G., *Grateful Memories: The Orthopaedic Hospital 1900–1988*, Oswestry, League of Friends of the Robert Jones and Agnes Hunt Orthopaedic Hospital, 1988

[22] Carter, M., *Healing & Hope*, Robert Jones and Agnes Hunt Orthopaedic and District NHS Trust, 2000

[23] Abrahams, G., *Grateful Memories: The Orthopaedic Hospital 1900–1988*, Oswestry, League of Friends of the Robert Jones and Agnes Hunt Orthopaedic Hospital, 1988

[24] Carter, M., *Healing & Hope*, op. cit.

[25] Ibid

[26] Ibid

[27] Hunt, Dame Agnes, *This is My Life*, London, Blackie, 1938

[28] Carter, M., *Healing & Hope*, op. cit.

[29] Hunt, *This is My Life*, op. cit.

Chapter 5
The School of Physiotherapy at Oswestry: 1920–1945

On the hospital's arrival at Park Hall, work was undertaken to make best use of the facilities of the site and to modify the original buildings to satisfy the needs of the new occupants. At an early stage in this remodelling, a new massage department was established, with direct access to the main corridor. It occupied approximately the same position as that of the physiotherapy department in the modern hospital. When the hospital first transferred from Baschurch, massage had been accommodated in a building not connected to the main corridor – a very unsatisfactory arrangement when it rained. The positioning of the new department enabled the majority of patients to be taken from the wards for treatment under the cover provided by a central corridor, a considerable improvement on the previous situation. Two years later, in 1924, a sunlight department was opened in a separate hut and a gymnasium was provided for more active rehabilitation of patients.[1]

These arrangements were a significant improvement on the cramped and outmoded buildings the hospital had occupied at Baschurch, but as a former student, Edna Longson, recalls, the realities of the hospital at Park Hall still left much to be desired and would not be acceptable today. Edna's impressions on arrival at Oswestry in 1923[2] identify the hospital as an extremely primitive place with the wards constructed from a series of prefabricated sheds which were open to the elements on one side. These wards were sun-scorched during the summer and quickly flooded when it rained. Counterpanes floated like magic carpets when the wind blew and snow seeped everywhere in winter. Students wore cardigans, gloves and fur boots to combat the cold but always suffered from chapped hands and chilblains.

During a time when the hospital was plagued by rats, one took up residence in a dressing room and others cavorted in the ward kitchens, defying the best efforts of the boilerman's cat to remove them. Students on night duty were particularly perplexed by the latter as they had to make frequent journeys to the ward kitchen to fill the bed warmers for the patients from a vat of water always kept on the boil. Despite all these adverse conditions, patients responded well to the excellent nursing care given and in time were cured of diseases such as tuberculosis of joints for which there was as yet no useful drug medication. Scrupulous attention was paid to sterility of instruments and dressings were changed and wounds cleared of infection without the aid of antibiotics.

The students' home was no less spartan than the wards, being unbearably hot in summer and exceedingly cold in winter when shoes froze to the floor and hair froze to the pillow while mice cavorted in the wardrobes. Students were obliged to be modest in dress when outside the hospital and wore long coats to cover their legs as their gymslips, although long by modern standards, displayed a few inches of leg and ankle, which was considered forward. Any houseman wishing to take a student out had first to receive permission from matron, who then stayed up to await the couple's return. History does not record if matron was aware of the many clandestine meetings on the theatre back porch, but she probably was and unobtrusively monitored those as well. Despite these hardships, the hospital was a happy place. Everyone worked hard and played harder. Tennis, golf and hockey occupied off-duty hours and, after the course studies were finished, student physiotherapists were taught to ride a motorcycle in preparation for work as aftercare sisters.

Dame Agnes believed in the healing power of fresh air and sunshine combined with inner cleanliness. Plentiful hot water cared for the former while a diet of prunes and rhubarb took care of the latter. Ward floors were scrubbed once a week by a team of ladies working on their hands and knees. It was rather like painting the Forth Bridge – a never-ending job.

The training arrangements for massage and remedial gymnastics also transferred to the Park Hall site with the rest of the hospital. The tutor, Miss Pearce, assisted by Miss Ewart, a remedial gymnast, was responsible for the education of students in these subjects. This partnership was, however, destined not to continue for long as, by 1923, both had left the hospital. Miss Ewart had resigned to take up a better-paid post on the staff of the Bergman Osterberg Physical Training College, Dartford Heath,[3] which closed in 1927 when the Conjoint Examination replaced single subject examinations for membership of the Chartered Society of Massage and Medical Gymnastics.[4]

In 1922, the Chartered Society of Massage and Medical Gymnastics (CSMMG) introduced the Conjoint Examination designed to replace the separate subject examinations in massage and medical gymnastics. Also in the same year, an association of teachers was established to provide a collective base for the sharing of knowledge and the support of new teachers entering the profession. This was one of the first specific interest groups within the CSMMG.[5] These developments in education stimulated hospital management to appoint staff specifically for the school of massage and, in August 1923, Miss Dalton was appointed principal. She remained the only qualified teacher on the staff until 1930 when she was joined by Miss P.M. Cooke,[6] a trained, certificated gymnast who was offered a salary of ninety pounds per annum all found.

Miss Dalton developed and implemented the new curriculum that was required for the preparation of candidates for the Conjoint Examination of the CSMMG. Initially students taking the Conjoint Examination worked alongside those already in training who were preparing for the separate subject examinations being phased out. By 1927, the Conjoint Examination was identified as the minimum requirement for membership of the CSMMG and schools continuing to prepare for single-subject examinations only were closed.

Although Miss Dalton was appointed principal, the School of Massage had no independence or autonomy as it was operated under the direct authority of the hospital matron, Miss Evelyn Murray. It was she who was responsible for the interview of candidates prior to admission to the combined course in orthopaedic nursing/massage and remedial gymnastics, who reported on their progress and discharged those who failed to meet the hospital's requirements. This situation continued until the 1960s, when student needs had changed, the two disciplines had diverged significantly and each profession had developed more sophistication in both its knowledge base and scope of professional practice.

To have established the hospital and developed orthopaedics as a highly specialised branch of the nursing profession, to have established also training for probationer nurses and masseuses, is a level of achievement that would have satisfied most people for a lifetime's endeavour. However, for Agnes, this was only the first phase of a multifaceted plan which she was able to develop fully during the 1920s. She ascribed totally to Ruskin's ideal of self-sufficiency for the disabled. Agnes recognised, partly as the result of her own experiences, that the most help she could ultimately give her patients was to make them useful to society, enabling them to earn a living rather than begging for it.

The second part of her plan was to establish a network of clinics, serviced by highly trained Oswestry staff, to review patients at regular intervals following their discharge from hospital. The purpose of these was to ensure that the progress made in hospital was maintained, splints were adjusted or replaced as required and families were compliant with and continuing the prescribed treatment regimes at home. This programme, named the Aftercare Service, was an instant success and provided much-needed support for patients and their families following their return home.

Being crippled presented major challenges to the majority of former patients who were unable to gain employment and so found it difficult to support themselves or their families. From the earliest days at Baschurch, Agnes had made use of patients' skills by encouraging them to do odd jobs around the hospital. In some cases, former patients had been trained in specific new skills – for example, lining with leather the splints and casts she had made to provide additional comfort to the wearer. Expanding on this idea, she founded, adjacent to the Oswestry hospital site, the Derwen Cripples Training College, where disabled people were given training in occupations such as cobbling and furniture restoration, which provided an income throughout their working lives. This was the final stage in the fulfilment of the ideal she had long held.

In 1923, Agnes Hunt's health had broken down once more and, for the next five years, periods of illness were interspersed with times when she was able to continue in her capacity as honorary superintendent at the hospital. Following her official retirement in 1928, she continued to visit the hospital almost daily and also retained a dominant position on all the committees concerned with operation and development of the hospital.[7] She was closely involved with the protracted negotiations for and the building of the new hospital to replace the original First World War Military Hospital accommodation into which the hospital had moved in 1921. This project finally got under way in the early 1930s[8] but was, unfortunately, halted by the outbreak of the Second World War when only half completed.

Qualified teachers of massage and medical gymnastics tended to work in very isolated situations. There were, at this time, numerous small schools of physiotherapy scattered about the country and frequently, as at Oswestry, there would be only one or at the most two qualified teachers working in an individual school. The Teachers' Association provided a useful forum for discussion and exchange of ideas. From its inception, the association organised courses and held conferences during university vacations to minimise interruption of the implementation of the curriculum teaching at the members' schools. Because of this arrangement, the Board of Management was able to support Miss Dalton's attendance at a course in Brighton in 1932, paying the lecture fee of two guineas and board and lodging charge of five pounds.[9]

By the late 1920s, discrepancies had arisen in student performance between the hospital examinations for the Orthopaedic Nursing Certificate and the CSMMG national examinations. A particularly striking example is observed by consideration of the November 1929 examination results. Of the twelve students who sat the CSMMG examinations, eleven passed and one failed the viva. Eight of the same students sat for the final orthopaedic nursing examination a short time afterwards, but, in this case, only three passed and five failed.

The Conjoint Examination of the CSMMG had been held in London and was recognised as being a taxing experience for all concerned. Members of the committee congratulated both the students and teachers on the satisfactory results achieved. They were concerned, however, that these same students had achieved such poor results in the hospital examinations held almost immediately afterwards, particularly as candidates had failed in orthopaedics and passed in anatomy.[10] The ensuing discussions were extensive and wide ranging, with all members of the committee expressing concerns, giving opinions, offering advice and generally considering the situation from an individual viewpoint without knowing the source of the discrepancy.

The future of the candidates who had failed the hospital examination was, unsurprisingly, left to matron's discretion, and it was she who discovered the explanation for the disparity of achievement by this group of students. They had studied hard for the CSMMG examinations and were rewarded by success. However, they admitted they had not studied significantly for the orthopaedic final examination, as they had heard that, on this occasion, Agnes Hunt was to be replaced as examiner by a doctor and, mistakenly, they considered this doctor would not fail them.[11]

Student perceptions were that it was very important for them to pass the CSMMG examinations at first attempt, as, in 1930, a regulation had been issued requiring candidates who failed a single examination component to retake all the subjects of the examination including those passed at the first attempt. This new regulation meant that candidates studying for resit examinations would need to devote all their energies to study between the two diets of the examination and would no longer be able to divide the time equally between nursing and study as they had prior to the new regulation.[12]

Electrical modalities were now being used extensively in patient treatment programmes across the country including those of the Shropshire Orthopaedic Hospital. However, although the scope of practice in this discipline was developing rapidly, it was not until 1929 that a CSMMG examination in medical electricity and light therapy was introduced. By the late 1930s, revision of the syllabus and amalgamation of the two subjects enabled candidates to gain a qualification in electrotherapy after following a training of seven months' duration. Electrotherapy is now recognised as the third core skill of physiotherapy practice; however, it remained the Cinderella service for many years, retaining a separate qualification until the late 1940s.[13]

Oswestry patients had been treated regularly with sunlight, galvanism and faradism since approximately 1915, but no official training had been offered to students in this area of practice. In 1929 the deficit was remedied when arrangements were made for two students to attend the course and take the CSMMG Certificate in Medical Electricity and Light Therapy offered by the Royal Southern Hospital in Liverpool. The Oswestry Board of Management supported the students by providing their board and lodging for the required four months of study. In return, students agreed to work at the Shropshire Orthopaedic Hospital for a further year, earning a salary of fifty pounds for their service. In the first year of operation of the scheme, four students qualified and proved to be extremely useful and valuable senior nurses and masseuses on their return to the hospital.[14] Following on this initial success, a further six students and an aftercare sister of five years' standing took the course in 1930.[15]

Although this association with the Royal Southern Hospital could be considered a success, it had significant limitations. Places on the Liverpool-based course could be offered to a limited number of students only and so training in this subject area was not available to all trainees from Oswestry. Dame Agnes reported to the hospital's Board of Management that the Certificate in Medical Electricity and Light Therapy was a prerequisite now demanded by all local authorities considering applicants for appointment as orthopaedic aftercare sisters. Applicants for these posts were at a disadvantage if they had trained at Oswestry, as the hospital could not provide the qualifications now expected. This was an unacceptable situation for the hospital that had developed the concept of aftercare and Agnes considered they would now be obliged to organise their own course in these subject areas.

Students were already being prepared for the Certificate in Orthopaedic Nursing offered by the hospital and the Certificate in Massage and Medical Gymnastics offered by the CSMMG. Training in medical electricity and light therapy was seen a natural and necessary development of the school's curriculum if it was to remain attractive to students applying to the hospital for training.[16]

Agnes was not a person to lose an opportunity for expansion of the hospital's portfolio of courses and she had already approached the Royal Salop Infirmary in Shrewsbury for its cooperation with the Board of Management of the Shropshire Orthopaedic Hospital to organise the additional training. Incorporation of this new subject into the existing course required considerable reorganisation. It was proposed that students would study at Oswestry for five years, spending two years nursing on the wards, followed by two years in the massage department, during which time students would enter the Conjoint Examination of the CSMMG and the Junior and Senior Orthopaedic Nursing Certificate examinations. This was to be followed by one year in special department work at a salary of forty pounds for the year.

Mr Lavall, a qualified radiologist in charge of the electrical room at the Royal Salop Infirmary, was prepared to undertake tuition of the Oswestry students provided he was paid for this additional responsibility. It was proposed students would travel to the Royal Salop Infirmary daily to attend lectures and treat patients under supervision between 09.00 and 13.00. The Oswestry hospital would also be required to appoint a qualified teacher in medical gymnastics and medical electricity, at a salary of £200 per annum to supervise student electrical practice at the hospital. Students would take the final examination in orthopaedic nursing during the fifth year of their course and it was suggested that, during the two years in the massage department, they should be given weekly lectures in orthopaedics to maintain their level of knowledge of the subject.[17]

This new scheme was an extension of the training provision already in place at the Shropshire Orthopaedic Hospital, but still required approval by the Chartered Society of Massage and Medical Gymnastics before it could be implemented. Progress on detailed negotiations with the Royal Salop Infirmary was delayed until the facilities offered had been inspected by a representative of the CSMMG.[18] The departments at the Royal Salop Infirmary and the Shropshire Orthopaedic Hospital were finally inspected in January 1932[19] and, in anticipation of a favourable report, Mr Lavall, Radiologist at the RSI, was appointed Radiologist and Lecturer in Medical Electricity and Light Therapy to the Massage School with an annual honorarium of £150.[20]

In order that the syllabus could be covered satisfactorily at the RSI, the CSMMG Representatives recommended the transfer of a spare carbon arc lamp from Oswestry to the RSI and purchase of a water-cooled mercury vapour lamp (Kromayer) for the Shrewsbury hospital. The thirty-six pounds cost of the new lamp was to be shared by the hospitals. About this time also, a teaching aid – an epidiascope – was purchased to assist the educational activities that were so much a part of the hospital's life, at a cost of thirty-seven pounds.[21]

The course in medical electricity, light therapy and diathermy arranged and organised with the RSI replaced arrangements for studies at the Royal Southern Hospital in Liverpool. Students were now required to pay five guineas for tuition and examination fees in return for the opportunity to gain the relevant CSMMG Certificate. The Board of Management of the Hospital agreed to provide students with free board, lodging and laundry for the duration of this additional component to the original course. Dame Agnes was very concerned that these arrangements might prove too costly for some students, making it difficult for them to complete the new qualification, and proposed that additional financial assistance was to be made available by the hospital for anyone proven to be in this untenable situation.[22]

By the end of the year, the first three students to complete the course had entered the examination in medical electricity and light therapy, but unfortunately, on this occasion, only one gained the Certificate.[23] During the same examination period, eleven students entered and passed the orthopaedic nursing finals and the CSMMG final examinations.

Concerns were now being expressed about the range of treatments practised by students. Oswestry continued to offer excellent experience in orthopaedics, but the hospital did not cater for patients who had been subjected to general surgery or suffered from medical conditions. A course of lectures on the treatment of medical conditions was organised and delivered by doctors based at the Royal Salop Infirmary and limited clinical experience had been gained by students on secondment to the Manchester Royal Infirmary. Unfortunately, it proved difficult to organise these secondments and it was impossible to continue with this particular attempt to increase the breadth of clinical experience for the Oswestry students.[24] During the mid 1930s, lectures on dissection were arranged for the students at the medical school at Birmingham University. The course, aimed to improve understanding of anatomy, also presented problems for the organisers and lasted a very short time. By the end of the decade, more permanent arrangements had been negotiated with Liverpool University.

There were changes in the status of the Orthopaedic Nursing Certificate around this time as a new ruling required all ward sisters appointed in a hospital to be qualified and registered general nurses. This had not always been the case at the Shropshire Orthopaedic Hospital as it was the individual's capability and experience in the specialised nursing and care of patients with orthopaedic conditions that was the guiding factor to appointment. Once the rule came into force, it became necessary to make formal arrangements with certain general hospitals to allow student nurses who had qualified from the Shropshire Orthopaedic Hospital to continue their studies for state registration in nursing. Their studies in orthopaedic nursing were credited by allowing entry to the general nursing course at affiliated hospitals at the post-preliminary stage, provided they had taken and passed the preliminary examinations in general nursing before leaving the Shropshire Orthopaedic Hospital.[25] Later in the decade, the Orthopaedic Nursing Certificate was organised as a nationally managed programme of learning,[26] replacing the local arrangements that had existed for a quarter of a century.

By the late 1930s, the pattern of courses at the hospital was established and stable, and students who undertook training during the late 1930s and 1940s paint a vivid picture of their stay in Shropshire. They were paid approximately twenty pounds per year all found and, during the first two years of nursing, the work was very hard physically, with only one half-day off-duty granted each week. Even this was forfeited if a nurse missed breakfast three times during any week or if the time off coincided with one of the two or three evenings during the week when lectures were arranged. When not working on the wards, afternoons were spent in the pursuance of lively games of hockey, rounders, tennis or taking bicycle rides through the lanes and byways around the hospital. Off-duty excursions out of the hospital grounds were subject to a curfew of 10 p.m., easily enforced as all were resident in the Nurses' Home.[27]

During the two years of nursing, students progressed from Junior Probationer – 'Queen of the Sluice' on entry to the course – to First Nurse – 'Sister's Right-hand Person' with significant responsibility for dressings, record-keeping and nursing the very sick. Two three-month periods were spent on night duty, one session during each year of the course.[28] This was followed by an eighteen-month course to complete certification as a masseuse/medical gymnast. Lectures were given in anatomy, physiology and pathology, and students also undertook practical work on patients. Anatomy studies were supplemented by a course at Liverpool Medical School for instruction on prosected limbs and the brain.

In June 1936, a young staff nurse, Mary Powell, came from her training school, the London Hospital, to undertake the post-registration certificate in orthopaedic nursing. She found, at interview, the general air of informality of the hospital, the sunshine, flowers and trees all around very seductive. After several years' training in London it looked like heaven. The patients were brown as berries and looked incredibly healthy. She came as a staff nurse, a 'Green B', and she comments that, although she found the theoretical component of the course sparse, the training she gained in the specialised area of orthopaedic nursing given by her peers and ward sisters was exemplary.[29]

Since her arrival at Oswestry, she had been aware of a group of staff who appeared to her to be very important. They wore very faded blue frocks and came into the dining room with plaster all over their shoes. They tended to sit together and read broadsheet newspapers after their meals. They were, of course, masseuses, and as training was also available at the hospital, Mary tentatively asked Miss Murray, the matron, if she would ever be considered for entry to the course. Miss Murray appeared to reject the notion out of hand. However, a week before the next course was due to start, Mary was offered a place. Although students did not pay tuition fees or board during the fifteen-month massage course, neither did they receive a salary. When offered the place, Mary had precisely three pounds in her Post Office savings account to pay all incidental expenses for the next fifteen months. Sister Hilda Arthur, who had been at the hospital since she entered as a probationer in 1923, and had risen through the ranks to be plaster room superintendent, saved the day by offering to lend Mary one pound a month when the three pounds had run out. This act of pure unselfish kindness enabled Mary Powell to qualify as a masseuse and eventually she reimbursed Hilda Arthur the sum of £13.[30]

Hilda Arthur's loan enabled Mary Powell to buy second-hand gym tunics and blouses, necessary for the daily classes in educational gymnastics that comprised mainly of the performance of 'long fly' over the horse. For this exercise, the gymnasium doors were held open and, if students gained sufficient speed on the approach to the horse, they could finish the long fly half way down Goodford Ward. Patients used to peep through the windows and note with pride, 'Look, there's my massage nurse,' as another student hurtled through the air. Other curriculum subjects were taught in a small classroom located by the physiotherapy department.

After gaining the further qualifications offered by Oswestry, Mary Powell left the hospital between 1940 and 1942 to work in Glasgow, then returned as assistant matron in charge of the Gredington Children's Annexe for the duration of the Second World War. After another break from Oswestry, she returned once more and from 1962 until her official retirement in 1974, served the hospital as matron and then principal nursing officer. An outstanding teacher, she was the author of the standard textbook on orthopaedic nursing, which ran to nine editions. She also lectured extensively in America and Australia and took the principles of Oswestry orthopaedic nursing to many distant countries such as Hong Kong, the Philippines, India and Burma.[31]

After almost two decades of uncertain peace, the storm clouds of another war were gathering over Europe. The Shropshire Orthopaedic Hospital quickly made its preparations, filled its sandbags, determined evacuation procedures in the event of attack and practised 'blacking out' the open-sided wards. There was an unexpected chance to prove the effectiveness of their plans when, on the evening the war started, a false alarm caused an air raid warning to be given in error. When the alarm sounded, all day staff returned to their posts immediately as planned and remained on duty in the darkened wards until the All Clear was given.[32]

Once again, the Shropshire Orthopaedic Hospital had a valuable role to play in a time of national crisis as it was graded a Base Hospital. During the First World War, the first group of military patients admitted to Baschurch were at a convalescent stage or were walking wounded. It was not long, however, before the hospital received severely wounded soldiers straight from the trenches. At the outbreak of the Second World War, the hospital was given the classification of Base Hospital and severely injured military patients were admitted to the hospital immediately on repatriation from the battlefields from the outbreak of the war. Wounded soldiers were often in the Oswestry Base Hospital within forty-eight hours of receiving their injuries. To accommodate the many wounded servicemen admitted, bed numbers were almost doubled, increasing from 360 to 715 between 1942 and 1945.[33]

Treatment of civilian patients continued for the duration of the war with adult patients remaining on the Gobowen site. Additional accommodation was provided to allow continuing care of children by the establishment of special annexes at Aston Hall, Oswestry, and at Gredington, Whitchurch, a facility provided by Lord Kenyon.[34] Not only was Gredington a facility for the treatment of children but also, prior to the final offensives of the war, the grounds were used for training manoeuvres by American servicemen preparing for the Normandy offensive. Sadly, after the landings had been made on Utah and Omaha beaches, many returned to a temporary hospital also built in the Gredington grounds, for treatment of injuries they had received in France.[35]

The high standards of orthopaedic work continued in the

annexes at Aston and Gredington, and, for students, the training was sound and effective, but the food was awful. Food rationing, the later stages of the war and coping with huge numbers of hungry young people by a cook who was used to the organised structured life of catering in a noble house conspired against the production of adequate, nourishing or interesting food. At Gredington, meals resembled those in a boarding school, with Sister Mary Powell presiding over the long refectory table. Giant aluminium trays were filled with dried egg powder and mixed with water. To this mixture, slices of cooked sausage were added and the whole was baked in the oven. When cooked, it was cut into squares, one for each person. Nurses and students sat down each side of the table, eking out the meagre portions of the boring repast to calm the pangs of their immediate hunger and dreaming of the slice of bread and syrup they would sneak from the ward kitchen on their return to duty.[36]

The electrotherapy component of physiotherapy was still a separate qualification and it was possible to be a qualified physiotherapist without having undertaken this additional training. However, in view of the well-heralded impending changes to the course to be implemented with the introduction of the National Health Service, Miss Dalton encouraged her pupils to complete their studies by taking courses in electrotherapy at either St Thomas' Hospital in London or at Glasgow Royal Infirmary. One student, Irene Addie,[37] recalls that she had been forbidden by her parents to go to London owing to the danger. Glasgow was considered to be the safer option. She was very pleased she had heeded this parental advice, when, during what would have been her first night at St Thomas', two wings of that hospital were razed to the ground with total destruction of the wards and departments they accommodated.

The course limped along in a relatively haphazard way with obviously less attention paid to student educational needs than to the care needs of the injured patients. Clinical caseloads were now expanded significantly to include the treatment of major trauma, fractures, ligament damage, nerve injuries and amputations. However, students continued to qualify from the school throughout the war years and shared particular experiences that fortunately have not been repeated on such a scale since it ended in 1945.

The first casualties to arrive at Oswestry after the evacuation from Dunkirk included one Czechoslovakian and a small number of Polish soldiers who had escaped to Britain. Another patient was a German airman whose plane had been shot down while on a bombing raid on Liverpool. He was not exactly popular with his fellow patients and, although under armed guard throughout his stay, continued to regale them with stories of Germany's superiority and the impending invasion of England by his countrymen. Many of the soldiers arrived at the hospital with severe infection to their wounds and great care had to be taken when changing dressings to limit the possibility of cross infection. Penicillin finally arrived, making a significant impact on the outcome of care packages towards the end of the conflict.

During their senior year, in addition to the long hours of ward duty, physiotherapy students worked a rotation for fire watching when the area was alerted to the possibility of an air raid. Three students were on duty at any one time and, in the event of the hospital being hit by a bomb, they were to alert all staff so that patients could be evacuated to the nearby hockey field and perceived safety. Fortunately, this never happened and the hospital escaped damage although, one night, incendiary bombs were dropped on the nearby Ruabon Hills by German planes returning home after a raid on Liverpool.[38] Vegetation ignited and the fire watchers were treated to the spectacle of a semicircular wall of flame illuminating the surrounding hills as they burned in the distance until dawn. These same students were attending dissection classes at the medical school in Liverpool and were able to see at first hand the terrible damage the raids inflicted on that city. Most recognisable landmarks had disappeared but, miraculously, the medical school escaped undamaged.[39]

Considerable hardship was experienced by the majority of the British population during the war years, strict food and clothing rationing compounded by the absence of choice among the limited stocks potential customers could find in the shops. No petrol was available for anything other than emergency use, so private cars were stored for the duration of the war. Garages and sheds were used to breed rabbits to supplement the tiny meat rations and every yard had its complement of hens to provide additions to the one egg per week allocated for each adult in the population. Even these meagre rations could not always be satisfied towards the end of the war and significant hardship was obvious. The Emergency Medical Service provided the food coupons and paid for the accommodation costs of treatment for the wounded servicemen, but civilian patients treated in the hospital were still funded solely by voluntary donation and contribution.

With the population worried and distracted by the events in Europe, students and staff were obliged to take every opportunity to remind people of the financial needs of the hospital and to boost its receipts. On one occasion, several probationer nurses/students were taken to a football match – technically an international as the teams represented Wales and England. During the half-time interval, loudspeaker announcements alerted the spectators to the necessity for financial support of the hospital while the probationers walked round the edge of the pitch near to the crowd, carrying grey army blankets, held by the corners, into which the spectators threw money. The crowd gave generously and, fortunately, as one of those probationers commented ruefully, no one required first aid, a subject not yet covered in their studies.[40]

Agnes had been created Dame Commander of the Order of the British Empire in 1926, two years before her official retirement and was, by the late 1930s, heavily involved with work for the Central Council for the Care of Cripples. She occupied the position of President during 1942,[41] travelling extensively throughout the country and pursuing the cause of the care of crippled children.

Now living in Selattyn, she retained her keen interest in all activities of the hospital. She was treated with great respect by everyone on her frequent visits and was always addressed as 'Sister' by the patients, staff and students she encountered. She still thought of the students as 'her children' although she no longer had any direct contact with them. Renowned for her kindness and generosity, she gave fruit or other garden produce to many of the wounded soldiers and spent much of her time with civilian patients, who received few visitors owing to the problems of transport. Nurses and students often used their afternoons off duty to cycle from the hospital to her home at Selattyn where they enjoyed the luxury of a boiled egg tea before returning to the hospital for further ward duty.[42]

The hospital was renamed after its founders in 1933, and, during the war, the Board of Management approached the College of Heralds for permission to develop a coat of arms for the hospital incorporating those of Sir Robert Jones and Dame Agnes Hunt respectively. The final design was developed with Sir Robert Jones' coat of arms on the left, with those of Dame Agnes on the right. The leopard's face is from the coat of arms of the County of Shropshire and the plant 'self-heal' has a special significance as it was one of the herbs used in the preparation of ointment used to anoint Our Lord's feet. The motto *Deo Dante Damus*, suggested by Lord Kenyon, translates to 'God gives that we may give to others'.

Permission was granted to use the armorial ensigns developed on seals and shields for use by the hospital and it was decided to incorporate the design in a badge to be offered to course qualifiers from the combined orthopaedic nursing and physiotherapy course. The first students to receive the badge qualified in 1944.[43]

After more than five years of austerity, conflict, excruciating hard work and uncertainty, the war came to an end in May 1945. The evening of the announcement, a student, concerned about the development of bunions had, during the day, 'borrowed' a pair of hallux valgus splints from the plaster room where she was working. These were about the size of the snowshoes worn by Inuits and Canadian trappers and quite similar in shape. A leather-lined metal sole plate with a straight medial border extended from the heel to a point beyond the end of the toes. The deviating great toe was strapped to the rigid metal to hold it in a straight position and other straps held the rest of the sole plate in place.

The student had just retired to bed when a tap on her door preceded the entry of Sister Mary Rowlands, the home sister, who whispered to her that the announcement of the end of the war had been made. Sister Rowlands then left and the student leapt out of bed to share the news with her friend and fell straight into her wardrobe as her feet were encased in the cumbersome hallux valgus splints.[44] No significant injuries were sustained, the splints were removed and the welcome news spread like wildfire around the hospital. Everyone danced and drank the night away in wild, uninhibited joy, releasing many of the tensions of the previous years. A bonfire was set alight on the ground outside the dining room and provided the focal point for the spontaneous festivities.

The following day, everyone poured out on to the playing fields; beds were decorated, staff wore fancy dress and toured the hospital grounds on floats which were, in reality, electric trolleys. Dame Agnes joined in the festivities, sharing her joy and relief with staff and patients of 'her' hospital.[45]

Once the war was over, military patients were discharged, either returning to their homes and families or transferring to hospitals and convalescent homes nearer to their families for further treatment. The separate annexes at Aston and Gredington were closed and the young patients who had spent the war years in these temporary quarters now returned to the main hospital base at Oswestry. On the surface, things appeared to be returning to normal. Finally, Evelyn Murray, matron of the hospital and Miss Dalton, principal of the school of physiotherapy, who had both extended their expected service to stay at the hospital until the war was over, retired and were replaced by Matron Bell and Miss Dorothy Talbot respectively.[46]

NOTES

[1] Carter, M., *Healing & Hope*, Robert Jones and Agnes Hunt Orthopaedic and District NHS Trust, 2000

[2] Longson (nee Taylor), E., student memories, 1923–1927

[3] Extracts from the minutes of the Committee of Visitors of the Shropshire Orthopaedic Hospital meeting, July 1923

[4] Chartered Society of Physiotherapy, '100 years 1894–1994', *Physiotherapy* vol. 80 issue A, 1994

[5] Chartered Society of Physiotherapy, '100 years 1894–1994', *Physiotherapy* vol. 80 issue A, 1994

[6] Extracts from the Minutes of the House Committee of the Shropshire Orthopaedic Hospital meeting, 18 September 1930

[7] Carter, M., *Healing & Hope*, Robert Jones and Agnes Hunt Orthopaedic and District NHS Trust, 2000

[8] Ibid

[9] Extracts from the minutes of the Board of Management of the Shropshire Orthopaedic Hospital meeting, 27 February 1932

[10] Extracts from the minutes of the House Committee of the Shropshire Orthopaedic Hospital meeting, 19 December 1929

[11] Ibid

[12] Extracts from the minutes of the House Committee of the Shropshire Orthopaedic Hospital meeting, 17 July 1930

[13] Chartered Society of Physiotherapy, '100 years 1894–1994', op. cit.

[14] Extracts from the minutes of the House Committee of the Shropshire Orthopaedic Hospital meeting, 18 September 1930

[15] Extracts from the minutes of the Board of Management of the Shropshire Orthopaedic Hospital meeting, 25 October 1930

[16] Extracts from the minutes of the Board of Management of the Shropshire Orthopaedic Hospital meeting held at Shrewsbury, 31 October 1931

[17] Extracts from the notes of a conference held at the Shropshire Orthopaedic Hospital, 26 October 1931

[18] Extracts from the minutes of the Board of Management of the Shropshire Orthopaedic Hospital meeting held at Shrewsbury, 28 November 1931

[19] Extracts from the report following the inspection of premises at the Royal Salop Infirmary and the Shropshire Orthopaedic Hospital by the Chartered Society of Massage and Medical Gymnastics, 28 January 1932

[20] Extracts from the minutes of the Medical Committee of Shropshire Orthopaedic Hospital meeting, 12 February 1932

[21] Extracts from the minutes of the House Committee of the Shropshire Orthopaedic Hospital meeting, 15 December 1932

[22] Extracts from the minutes of the Board of Management of the Shropshire Orthopaedic Hospital meeting, 19 March 1932

[23] Extracts from the minutes of the House Committee of the Shropshire Orthopaedic Hospital meeting, 15 December 1932

[24] Extracts from the minutes of the House Committee of the Shropshire Orthopaedic Hospital meeting, 28 January 1932

[25] Extracts from the minutes of the Examination Board of the Shropshire Orthopaedic Hospital, 11 December 1931

[26] Rowe (nee Bolton), K.E., student memories, 1936–1941

[27] Ibid

[28] Ibid

[29] Powell, M., student memories, 1936–1941, Journal of the Old Oswestrian Physiotherapists Association, 1958–1959

[30] Ibid

[31] *The Heritage of Oswestry – The origin and development of the Robert Jones and Agnes Hunt Orthopaedic Hospital, Oswestry, 1900–1975,* Oswestry, The Robert Jones and Agnes Hunt Orthopaedic Hospital, 1975

[32] Rowe, student memories, op. cit.

[33] Carter, M., *Healing & Hope*, Robert Jones and Agnes Hunt Orthopaedic and District NHS Trust, 2000

[34] Ibid

[35] Roberts, H., student memories, 1943–1948

[36] Ibid

[37] Addie, I., student memories, 1939–1944

[38] Linklater (nee Knight), B., student memories, 1943–1948

[39] Ibid

[40] Gardner, M., student memories, 1943–1948

[41] Extracts from the Supplement to Newsletter no. 11, British Orthopaedic Association, July 1942

[42] Gardner, M., student memories, 1943–1948

[43] Menzies, J.C., Journal of the Old Oswestrian Physiotherapists' Association, 1956–1957

[44] Alexander, A., student memories, 1943–1948

[45] Roberts, H., student memories, 1943–1948

[46] Extracts from minutes of the Board of Management of the Robert Jones and Agnes Hunt Orthopaedic Hospital meeting, 16 August 1945

Chapter 6
Preparing for the National Health Service:1942–1948

Approximately halfway through the war the hospital was battling with the enormous workloads generated by the care of over 700 patients scattered over three main sites. Staff suffered significant personal privations as a consequence of a conflict of this magnitude and all were uncertain as to the final outcome of hostilities. Into this overcharged, strained situation, the Beveridge Report was received and caused yet further concern about the future and viability of the hospital.

Sir William Beveridge, the author of the report, had worked with the Government in the field of social reform both before and during the First World War. At the outbreak of the Second World War, he again indicated his willingness to serve his country and on this occasion was offered the chairmanship of a committee enquiring into the coordination of the social services. The committee was expected to present its findings once the war was ended, but within eighteen months, late in 1942, the Beveridge Report[1] was published. The general public were ecstatic about the contents of the report and, by applying pressure on Parliament, forced the apathetic government reluctantly to accept it.

The most important issue in the report was the proposal for introduction of a nationalised health care system once the war ended. By this time, the Robert Jones and Agnes Hunt Orthopaedic Hospital had reached a peak of excellence in orthopaedic care, recognised throughout the world. The new National Health Service appeared nonplussed by such a high level of expertise in a relatively narrow field as its objective was primarily to provide a level of competent healthcare over the whole spectrum of need rather than lauding the high level of expertise in such a 'specialist' centre. How and where the hospital would fit in with the new arrangements gave rise to long debate by the Board of Management, but slowly, as the government's plans unfurled, hospital personnel came to terms with the broad principles of the proposed scheme.

The establishment of a comprehensive health service designed to secure general improvement in the physical and mental health of the population and the prevention, diagnosis and treatment of illness became the responsibility of the new Minister of Health. A government White Paper, published in 1944, identified that services were, in the main, to be provided free of charge and supplied on the basis of need rather than on the ability to pay. Subsequently, the proposals contained in the Beveridge Report formed the basis of the National Health Services Act (1946) and the system was launched two years later.

The new centrally funded service also took responsibility for education of some of the professional groups involved in patient care, including doctors, nurses and physiotherapists. Financial requirements of these educational activities were to be identified centrally, then cascaded downwards to the point of delivery. The finance supporting medical and nurse education was ring-fenced at source, protected as it passed down through the tiers of administration, earmarked for specific use by the institutions providing nurse training and clinical training of doctors. Funding for physiotherapy education was also determined centrally, but as it was not ring-fenced, once cascaded to regional level, it was no longer identifiable. Without the protection afforded by ring-fencing, financial support of physiotherapy courses became a lottery, in which schools competed with all other regionally financed services for a share of ever-dwindling resources. As school personnel were not directly involved in patient care, they fared badly in the allocation of monies, gradually falling far behind schools of nursing in the level of provision of equipment, staffing levels and other services required by their students.

In 1943, the Chartered Society of Massage and Medical Gymnastics changed its name once more to become the Chartered Society of Physiotherapy (CSP)[2] and evaluated its syllabus of training to determine if it still prepared students to meet the current demands in the workplace. It was then obvious that a major review of the curriculum was required and this was undertaken between 1943 and 1947. As a result of this review, the society's training was extended to three years and two months under the overall title of 'physiotherapy'. Previously, the course had prepared candidates for practice in massage and medical gymnastics, encompassing manipulation and movement, two of the three core skills of physiotherapy. Electrotherapy, the third core skill, had remained a separate qualification and it was not compulsory to train in this subject area until the introduction of the new CSP syllabus which coincided with the start of the NHS. The incorporation of electrotherapy, the profession's third core skill, into the basic curriculum of the Chartered Society, allowed the introduction in 1948 of a single qualification for successful candidates of membership of the Chartered Society of Physiotherapy (MCSP).[3] It was identified also that students would, under the new curriculum, receive not less than three weeks' nursing experience and spend a minimum of 750 hours during the course treating patients, guided by qualified staff of the department.

The curriculum review had been triggered by developments in physiotherapy practice and also by publication, in May 1944, of the Goodenough Report[4] which had enquired into the organisation and future of medical education. The report had laid down guidelines for medical education in the UK which were to be followed for the next forty years, and this helped the CSP curriculum reviewers to bring physiotherapy education more into line with other medically based courses. Preparation for a career in physiotherapy was considered to be a graduated educational process culminating in professional qualification and, although schools were hospital-based, the first year of the course could be located in a university.[5] It was, however, to be nearly fifty years before this ideal became a reality and all UK schools of physiotherapy were relocated as university departments.

The syllabus to be examined consisted of anatomy, physiology, massage, movement, physics, electrotherapy, patient care and medical and surgical conditions treated by physiotherapy. Studies in psychology, ethical laws and professional etiquette were also required and it was expected that the principles of rehabilitation would be taught related to all treatments. Courses were examination-orientated with relatively rigid regimes of physiotherapeutic techniques being applied to predetermined pathological states, the theory of which had been previously taught.

The assessment system was also revised and followed the Goodenough medical model as students came to accept examinations at eighteen, thirty and thirty-six months of the course. At eighteen months, the Preliminary examination consisted of three papers, one on physical principles and two on anatomy and physiology, supplemented by a viva of fifteen minutes. At thirty months, students sat the Intermediate examination. With three papers and three practical examinations this was a major hurdle at which many a student fell in at least one component. There was a paper on the theory and techniques of massage, movement and electrotherapy and two more on the treatment of patients by physiotherapy. All papers in both the Preliminary and Intermediate examinations were three hours long and required essay-style answers to the questions posed.

The practical element of the Intermediate examination consisted of thirty-minute assessments of the skills of massage, movement (including group exercise) and electrotherapy. Models for all examinations were junior physiotherapy students who were coerced into 'volunteering' on the understanding it was a good learning experience.

Once the Intermediate examination was over, the Final examination came at the end of the course. It lasted for two hours, during which time the candidate demonstrated the physiotherapeutic management of three 'cases'. Success in this examination depended significantly on the models' ability to maintain the behaviours and symptoms of, for example, patients following a 'stroke', suffering from an osteoarthritic hip or possibly acting as a child with a form of cerebral palsy.[6] Throughout this proposed new scheme, students were trained to recognise a pattern of symptomology to which they applied a predetermined treatment schedule. It was to be many years before students were educated to assess patient problems and apply deductive reasoning to determine strategies for maximal therapeutic benefit in a programme of rehabilitation.

The launch of this revised curriculum and examination system was planned to coincide with the introduction of the National Health Service in 1948. Schools that wished to continue to offer courses culminating in membership of the Chartered Society of Physiotherapy were required not only to offer their students adequate teaching in electrotherapy but also access to the treatment of patients suffering from the full range of conditions normally treated by physiotherapy.

Dame Agnes, still a powerful voice on all the hospital committees, was more concerned with preserving the integrity of the training she had developed than she was in conforming to the new, generalist requirements for physiotherapy pre-registration education proposed by the CSP. The original combined training in orthopaedic nursing and physiotherapy offered by the hospital had been developed specifically to satisfy specific patient needs. Initially patients were treated in hospital and then, with establishment of the Aftercare Service, continuing expert supervision was provided for patients once they had been discharged from hospital and returned to their homes. Prior to the introduction of the NHS, the Oswestry School of Massage and Medical Gymnastics was at the height of its success and if it had closed then would have been remembered with pride for its pioneering work in orthopaedic physiotherapy and initiation of Aftercare Services.

The hospital's Board of Management, after long discussion, came to the conclusion that the hospital would not be able to satisfy the additional demands of the new CSP curriculum and initially considered closing the school. However, as closure would have a major negative impact on future staff recruitment, the committee was urged to reconsider their options and find an alternative solution.

The next consideration was to continue the existing course at Oswestry with the addition of electrotherapy to the curriculum. With this slight alteration to the course, it was hoped to continue the training of specialist orthopaedic aftercare sisters. It was anticipated they would be eligible for associate membership of the CSP as the course they would have followed would not have included the required amount of general experience prior to qualification, for full membership of the CSP. As expected, discussion of this possibility continued for many months with little realistic progress being made. However, it transpired that associate membership, once considered by the CSP as a solution for the courses offered by 'specialist hospitals' such as Oswestry, had fallen into logistical difficulties over definition and had been withdrawn. For some time after receiving this unwelcome news, the members of the relevant hospital committees avoided further discussion of this particularly irritating problem and devoted their full energies to the care of their many patients, hoping the war would end before these energies were totally depleted.

There had been sporadic intermittent correspondence between the government and the CSP considering the hospital's position in relation to implementation of the proposed new course. At one stage, Matron Murray and 'Sister Tutor', the principal of the school, Miss Dalton, were nominated to represent the school (based in a 'specialist hospital') to work on the new curriculum with the Chartered Society of Physiotherapy.[7]

The hospital had expanded dramatically during the war years and there were, by 1944, significantly increased numbers of potential physiotherapy students among the ranks of probationer nurses once they had completed their ONC studies. It was admitted with some reluctance that classroom size and staffing levels had remained unaltered despite these additional numbers and these were now inadequate to cope with course teaching in a peace-time environment.[8] Eventually, hospital management was forced to accept that the teaching of light and medical electricity, major components of the electrotherapy syllabus, presented no major problems if the hospital was prepared to purchase the necessary additional apparatus and appoint qualified teachers of the subject to implement the new programme. There was, however, no easy solution to the CSP requirement for student exposure to patients with medical and respiratory conditions in addition to the excellent orthopaedic experience they presently gained.[9]

By October 1944, the Board of Management had accepted that adaptation of the curriculum to include electrotherapy was a possibility and would become a practical proposition if the hospital were to be considered as a centre for the treatment of rheumatic disorders in the new health service. The hospital would be required to develop a specialist unit for long-stay rheumatic cases and these 'medical' patients would need significant physiotherapy care using all available modalities.[10] This would address in part the CSP requirement for the additional range of clinical exposure required to satisfy the new curriculum.

The Chartered Society of Physiotherapy had already indicated they did not mind how the proposed new syllabus of an individual course was organised, provided all required elements were covered and a further committee was constituted in the hospital to discuss the school's future.[11] Matters then appeared to move more quickly with the formation of this special subcommittee, consisting of Major Bury, Dr Taylor, the matron and two members of the Medical Committee. As the main function of the subcommittee was to consider the new syllabus of training suggested by the CSP, it is unfortunate that Miss Dalton, the principal of the school, was not invited to attend. She was the only person in the hospital with the specific knowledge required to organise the syllabus.

The Chartered Society had given almost five years' advance warning of the changes in the physiotherapy training courses and had offered advice and support to all schools. This was of particular importance to institutions such as Oswestry, where specific expertise was taught to a very high standard, but the full range of clinical experience required was not available. One of the solutions proposed by the CSP was for students training in these specialist schools to spend the last year in a general hospital in order to gain experience in treating cases not catered for in the parent hospital. Miss Dalton represented the Oswestry School at meetings with the CSP to discuss application and implementation of the proposed new syllabus and it was considered an agreement would have to be made with a general hospital for student exchanges to provide an adequate range of general experience.

Matters came to a head when it was finally realised the new curriculum would have to be introduced in all schools not later than September 1947. Junior nurses entering training at Oswestry in 1944 would, under the existing course arrangements, be eligible for the Massage course in 1947. Unless the electrotherapy curriculum was ready to be implemented at the hospital, these students would not be able to enter the new CSP Preliminary examination in May 1949.[12]

At last the war was now over and Miss Dalton, exhausted by all the additional problems caused by the proposed new curriculum, retired on 1 June 1945.[13] Miss Dorothy Talbot was appointed to succeed her and took up the post of principal on 1 September 1945.

Miss Talbot appeared to students to be a very young appointee, although she must have been in her thirties at the time. She was quiet, sober in dress and manner, and gave the impression, from first meeting, that there was a very active mind behind her ordinary appearance. In temperament, she was a gentle, kindly person who, despite her shyness, worked without rest for the school. She was assisted by her friend Elsa John, a talented artist, whose exquisite anatomical drawings compensated for the lack of illustrated texts available in immediate post-war months and are remembered well by students at the time.[14]

Dorothy Talbot adapted quickly to her new role as principal of the school as students returned to the familiar routine of lectures, ward work and examinations, hockey in the afternoon and chapel in the evening. Within months of her appointment, she had considered all the possibilities for the school's continuance within the NHS that her predecessors had explored. She accepted that the course designed had to satisfy the requirements of the new CSP syllabus if the school were to be incorporated into the NHS. It became Miss Talbot's top priority to find a permanent solution. The first area she addressed was the teaching of electrotherapy. She agreed to teach this subject, suggesting that the existing syllabus be continued initially with the intake restricted to ten, owing to the limited equipment available for student practice. Students would be able to gain appropriate clinical experience in Wrexham. Confirmation of her appointment to the post of principal and approval of the proposals for implementation of the electrotherapy course would be granted following an inspection by the Chartered Society of Physiotherapy.[15]

This inspection was carried out on 5 December 1945 and the visitors obviously enjoyed their visit. One of them, Dr Lackenau, offered to come to Oswestry from London for two periods of three days each year to give additional electrotherapy lectures. The visitors were impressed by the confident manner with which students treated their patients, but concern was expressed by the lack of medical cases in the hospital and, on interviewing students who had just completed the course, this was considered to have been a disadvantage in the Final examinations. Miss Bartlett, the principal of the Liverpool School, was also one of the visitors and raised the possibility of student exchanges between the two schools. This would give Oswestry the opportunity to increase the range of clinical experience available to students.

Miss Talbot, with great energy and zeal, explored all reasonable possibilities for increasing the range of clinical experience in venues not too distant from Oswestry. Wrexham, Shrewsbury and other nearby hospitals were found to be lacking in both the range and quality of experience available and, finally, after much evaluation and negotiation, a full affiliation scheme was considered between the Wolverhampton Royal Hospital and the Robert Jones and Agnes Hunt Orthopaedic Hospital. The Royal Hospital at Wolverhampton was keen to train physiotherapists, but had neither the knowledge nor the resources to establish a school without significant assistance. They did, however, promise to support Oswestry students and undertook to provide the wide range of medical and surgical conditions required to balance Oswestry students' experience prior to entry to the Final CSP examinations. Wolverhampton would also benefit from the excellence of the orthopaedic experience available at Oswestry.

It was suggested the proposed school should open in September 1948, with biannual intakes of sixteen to twenty students. Some of these would have already completed the Orthopaedic Nursing Certificate; others would be direct entrants. Students who had already gained the ONC at Oswestry would spend eighteen months of the three-year physiotherapy course in Wolverhampton, six months in the preliminary training school and twelve months working part-time in the hospital physiotherapy department and clinics. They would then return to the RJAH to complete their studies. Students entering the course directly to Wolverhampton would spend the whole course there. If any direct entrant to the physiotherapy course subsequently wished to take the specialist orthopaedic course, it would be arranged. Wolverhampton had been approved for acceptance of candidates of both sexes as they wished to increase the opportunities for young men to train for physiotherapy.

Initially four qualified teachers would be required at Wolverhampton; three – Miss Talbot, Miss John and a teacher of electrotherapy, Miss Marriot – would be loaned by Oswestry for eighteen months to launch the scheme, and one teacher would be appointed directly by the Royal Hospital, Wolverhampton. Two classrooms would be provided, one for theory, the other for practical classes. Oswestry also agreed to loan to Wolverhampton furniture and technical equipment to ease the costs of implementation of the scheme.

Students were a valuable part of the workforce and any department supporting pre-registration clinical training calculated their staffing needs and then reduced their requirement by one qualified physiotherapist for each four students accommodated by the department. The proposed transfer to Wolverhampton for eighteen months of the course necessitated the appointment at Oswestry of four additional physiotherapists to compensate for the lost student work contribution. Correspondingly, Wolverhampton would require fewer qualified staff to service the departments once students were directly involved in patient treatments.[16]

Wolverhampton was as enthusiastic about the affiliation as was Oswestry, and both undertook to do everything in their power to make the joint school venture a success. Planning for the proposed affiliated school continued until the CSP inspection of the Wolverhampton facilities by Miss Owtram on 5 March 1948 when there was full discussion of all aspects of the proposal. Miss Owtram was satisfied with what she saw and indicated she would send a favourable report to the Training and Registration Committee of the CSP. The expected starting date for the new school was September 1948.[17] In the event, due to circumstances beyond their control, the school start date was retarded by four months and students were not admitted until January 1949.[18]

Notes

[1] Beveridge, W., *Social Insurance and Allied Services*, Cmd. 604, HMSO, 1942

[2] Chartered Society of Physiotherapy, '100 years 1894–1994', *Physiotherapy* vol. 80 issue A, 1994

[3] Tidswell, M., 'Physiotherapy: A True Profession?', unpublished MA dissertation, 1991

[4] Goodenough, *The Organisation and Future of Medical Education in the UK*, 1944

[5] Tidswell, 'Physiotherapy: A True Profession?', op. cit

[6] Chartered Society of Physiotherapy, '100 years 1894–1994', op. cit.

[7] Extracts from the minutes of the Board of Management meeting of the Robert Jones and Agnes Hunt Orthopaedic Hospital, 20 April 1944

[8] Extracts from the minutes of the Board of Management meeting of the Robert Jones and Agnes Hunt Orthopaedic Hospital, 20 July 1944

[9] Extracts from the minutes of the Board of Management meeting of the Robert Jones and Agnes Hunt Orthopaedic Hospital, 17 February 1944

[10] Extracts from the minutes of the Board of Management meeting of the Robert Jones and Agnes Hunt Orthopaedic Hospital, 19 October 1944

[11] Extracts from the minutes of the Board of Management meeting of the Robert Jones and Agnes Hunt Orthopaedic Hospital, 21 December 1944

[12] Extracts from the minutes of the Board of Management meeting of the Robert Jones and Agnes Hunt Orthopaedic Hospital, 15 February 1945

[13] Extracts from the minutes of the Board of Management meeting of the Robert Jones and Agnes Hunt Orthopaedic Hospital, 15 March 1945

[14] Roberts, H., student memories, 1943–1948

[15] Extracts from the minutes of the Board of Management meeting of the Robert Jones and Agnes Hunt Orthopaedic Hospital, 15 November 1945

[16] Extracts from the minutes of the Board of Management meeting of the Robert Jones and Agnes Hunt Orthopaedic Hospital, 19 December 1947

[17] Extracts from the minutes of the Board of Management meeting of the Robert Jones and Agnes Hunt Orthopaedic Hospital, 18 March 1948

[18] Extracts from the minutes of the Board of Management meeting of the Robert Jones and Agnes Hunt Orthopaedic Hospital, 17 October 1948

Chapter 7
A Year of Change: 1948

The evening of Tuesday, 27 January 1948 was cold, wet and miserable. The day it followed had been dreary and damp, typical of winter in Shropshire. A physiotherapy student and her army officer boyfriend walked to nearby Gobowen once they had both finished their day's duties[1] and by 8.30 p.m. were sitting in the Cross Keys public house, enjoying a drink, when they heard the sound of a fire alarm. Curious but unconcerned, they left the public house and walked a few yards down the road to Gobowen Station and climbed on to an iron bridge that spanned the railway line until the late 1970s. From this raised viewing point, the precise location of the fire was clearly identifiable to the couple. It was the hospital that was ablaze and not the nearby army camp as had been suspected. They rushed back to the hospital to witness the raging conflagration enveloping most of the hospital buildings, the flames fanned by the wind.

The fire had started in the dispensary and spread rapidly along the roof of the 720-foot-long corridor.[2] The roof spaces of all departments and the wards were continuous with that of the central corridor, providing a conduit for the fire to spread rapidly throughout the hospital.[3] At an early stage, it had taken a strong hold on the physiotherapy department, particularly the electrical treatment room and the students' classroom that contained all the electrical apparatus, books, student records, gymnastic and other equipment owned by the school. The buildings were at the end of the corridor next to the dispensary. Access to these two rooms was normally gained from the corridor and there was also an alternative entrance away from the flames. The keys to this other door were, however, kept in an office that was, by this time, at the heart of the fire. One of the physiotherapy students, with great courage and no consideration for her own safety, managed to enter the burning department by climbing the outside wall and breaking a window to gain access to the building. Once inside, she could see nothing as the electrical power had been lost and smoke obscured what little vision she would have had from other natural light sources. She felt her way carefully across the room towards a bolted door she knew was situated on the side of the building away from the fire. Once she had found the door, it took moments only to unbolt it and then several of her colleagues rushed in to the burning building and started emptying the classrooms.

The first item to be rescued was the school's prized articulated skeleton and then a heavy display cabinet containing beautifully mounted anatomical joints. Students and staff then pushed the majority of the electrical apparatus out of the burning building to safety. As they were clearing the room, the ceiling panels were burning through and dropping on to the floor all around them. Thankfully and surprisingly, these anonymous heroines all escaped unscathed and no one was injured that night. Once the electrical equipment, including a new short wave diathermy machine, had been moved to safety, rescuers eased their way into the classroom and managed to clear it of the remainder of the furniture, mainly desks and chairs. They were now being helped by numerous volunteers from Park Hall camp and between them they salvaged twenty out of the twenty-one desks, complete with books that had been in the classroom.[4]

The fire was moving with great speed up the corridor and was eventually controlled by a 'cordon sanitaire', created by destroying the corridor for a distance of approximately ten feet about the level of the present Concert Hall. Departments were emptied in advance of the flames; patient records, X-rays and the contents of the operating theatre were lodged on the playing fields together with the electrical equipment, skeleton and desks taken from the school.

At the same time, staff, volunteers, students and army personnel were evacuating wards and transporting patients to safety away from the flames. Beds and wheelchairs were pushed down the Burma Road by the light of an occasional torch, to Park Hall Camp where a 'spider' had been vacated for the displaced patients.

Many others were taken a few hundred yards along the road to the Derwen Cripples Training College. Aston Hall, the Children's Annexe, about three miles distant from the hospital, received approximately sixty children, complete with frames and splints, ferried there by car, lorry and ambulance from Oswestry. By 11 p.m., the hospital had been fully evacuated and the patients all found temporary accommodation.[5] One person only was not accounted for until, with a flash of inspiration, one of the exhausted firefighters called at the patient's house on his way to his own home. The patient's family had seen the flames from their house and had rushed over to the hospital, fought through the confusion to find their relative and had then pushed his bed three miles to the safety of his home.

The following morning, when Dame Agnes was informed of the disaster, her first concern was for the safety of the patients. On being assured that no patient nor member of staff had been injured by the fire although about half the hospital buildings had been destroyed, she said in a lighthearted manner that she had never liked the design of the new wards anyway and would not mourn their destruction. Not only were the physiotherapy, electrotherapy and ultraviolet light departments destroyed, but the hospital lost also its dental surgery, hospital library, linen store, pathology laboratory, students' lecture room, hospital stores, the main kitchen, Goodford, Kenyon, Gladstone and Wrekin wards, the teachers' room and the staff dining room.

With no classroom to use and no department in which to work, students were released from study to help ward staff return some semblance of order to the damaged hospital. The afternoon after the fire, students trawled through the ashes of the physiotherapy department with sticks, calliper irons or shovels, searching for all the metal hooks, rings and pulleys that would have survived the fire. Approximately seventy-five per cent of the original metal pieces were recovered from the charred remains of the department. They were cleaned, new ropes attached to the pulley blocks, and the hospital sewing room made sets of canvas slings and many sandbags of different weights. By these means, some of the suspension and gymnastic apparatus lost in the fire was able to be replaced with speed and at minimal cost.[6]

A week after the fire, Miss Talbot wrote to the Council of the Chartered Society of Physiotherapy detailing temporary arrangements she had made to enable the physiotherapy course to continue at Oswestry. She requested permission to complete the training of the two sets of students following the old CSMMG syllabus and the Conjoint Examinations who were due to qualify in May and November 1948. It had previously been arranged that, after September 1948, all teaching staff would move to Wolverhampton for eighteen months to start teaching the new CSP syllabus in the affiliated school, before returning to Oswestry in May 1950 to continue the course with their students.

At the time of writing this letter, a temporary physiotherapy department was under construction and would provide two treatment areas, each of them seventy feet long by twenty feet wide. Most of the department/school's electrical apparatus had been saved and suspension equipment replacement was in hand. Two huts in the hospital grounds had been offered as temporary replacement theoretical and practical classrooms and students would have use of the gymnasium at the Derwen Cripples Training College. As the physiotherapy department had been destroyed, all patient treatments were at that time being given on the wards, but it was hoped the new temporary department would be usable in a fortnight and finished within a month. Only one week's instruction of students had been lost as a result of the devastation of the hospital by the fire.[7]

The window ends of Goodford and Kenyon wards were brick built and were left standing after the fire. It was decided to use these ward ends to help construct a temporary physiotherapy unit. Within three weeks, the open sides of the wards had been covered in, partitions erected, walking bars and steps installed, the whole area furnished with borrowed or rescued furniture and an overhead pulley system put in place for the support of severely paralysed polio patients during exercise sessions.[8]

All records of students who had entered the school since it started in 1909 were lost in the fire. This posed no problems for physiotherapists who had already qualified, but for the students due to take final examinations in May and November there was great concern. As the professional organisation, the CSP, implemented the examination system, records of student achievement in the professional examinations were held centrally. Lost in the fire were hospital records of assessment of clinical competence, internal test results and any other information held on students. Over many evenings, Miss John and Miss Talbot worked to reconstruct these essential files to permit their students access to the Final examination as scheduled. The school managed to limp through this crisis, the examinations were taken on schedule and life for the moment appeared to settle down to its former routine.

The next event of this momentous year was the introduction of the NHS on 5 July, which came into being after years of planning, negotiating and preparing for the event. After nearly half a century of independent operation as a voluntary hospital, dependent on the generosity and careful financial management by a small band of dedicated people, the hospital became, on 5 July, the responsibility of a new Hospital Management Committee and the Birmingham Regional Hospital Board. By virtue of the quality of people involved with its management in these early transitional days, it became apparent that the pioneering spirit and the sense of purpose throughout the hospital would prevail in the new nationalised structure of health care provision.

Later in the month, on 25 July, Dame Agnes died. Coming so soon after the start of the NHS, it must have galvanised the new committees of management of the hospital to work harder to ensure her ideals were honoured and the 'spirit' of Oswestry preserved. Throughout her long life she had revolutionised the care of cripples, 'invented' orthopaedic nursing, started a school of physiotherapy, created the aftercare service and developed the Derwen Cripples Training College, where disabled youngsters learned the skills of an occupation that would provide financial independence throughout their working lives. She altered the country's attitude to and treatment of the disabled in a more significant way than has any other person before or since. Her partnership with Robert Jones was the deciding factor that determined the development of this internationally recognised and respected orthopaedic hospital. The alternative was to have continued as a kindly, well-meaning gentle institution providing convalescent care to a limited number of children in a smallish house in a quiet Shropshire village.

Students and staff continued to work towards the completion in November 1948 of the last of the courses to follow the now superseded syllabus and Conjoint Examinations. Arrangements were finalised for the temporary transfer of all the school's teaching to the Wolverhampton Royal Hospital for the start of the affiliated school in September. Premises there were made ready, furnished and equipped. At Oswestry, additional qualified staff were recruited to undertake the work normally undertaken by the students who were to be absent from the wards during the whole of 1949 and the early part of 1950. In making these calculations for additional staff, the work input of four students was equated to that expected of one qualified physiotherapist.

The transfer of teaching to the new affiliated school was, however, to be delayed by another catastrophe that hit the hospital in September 1948. Hazel Roberts, one of the students who had taken the Final examination in May 1948 had remained at the hospital on qualification to complete her service commitment to the hospital.[9] She describes graphically the air of depression that settled over the hospital as the staff sick bay in the Nurses' Home was filled with staff displaying flu-like symptoms, some of whom appeared to be rather ill.

The atmosphere of gloom and foreboding was heightened by the increasing size of the sick bay as more rooms were commandeered for use and the frequent comings and goings of senior hospital personnel, all wearing very worried expressions.[10] Staff received the first indication of the precise nature of the illness in an article that appeared in the *Border Counties Advertiser* on 13 October which reported that typhoid fever had been diagnosed in a number of staff on 10 September. There followed months of repeated screening and testing until all the victims of the disease had been found, isolated and treated. In all, it is thought there were 112 cases, but, as diagnosed typhoid sufferers were transferred to numerous small fever hospitals throughout Shropshire and the West Midlands, it is difficult to get accurate information about their care or the outcome of the disease process once they left the orthopaedic hospital. The source of the initial infection was never confirmed despite rigorous testing of all water supplies, sanitation, staff and patients. Once the problem had been identified, all resources were used to eradicate it effectively and speedily.

Staff continued their work schedules and regular testing, dreading the notification of a positive blood test result. One of the later victims of the disease was Hazel Roberts, who had qualified as a chartered physiotherapist and was in the final weeks of completion of her service obligation to the hospital when she received the news she had dreaded.[11] The official notification by telephone call came towards the end of the outbreak, when hope of escape from infection by the disease was beginning to permeate through the remaining staff. Sister Rowlands, the home sister, was the bearer of the news and organised Hazel's transfer to sick bay in a very practical manner. Hazel was instructed to go to her room and return to sick bay carrying her mattress, nothing else. The journey from room to sick bay was one of horror and shame; people encountered on the way recognised the bare mattress and knew what had transpired. They gave no encouragement or even a greeting, just cowered away from her as far as the narrow corridors would allow, for fear of contamination. People diagnosed with typhoid fever were isolated and alone, experiencing first hand the level of despair felt by lepers in earlier times. On arrival at sick bay, she was put to bed and left alone to wait for the next ambulance for transport to a fever hospital for treatment. The only personal possession allowed was a handbag, guarded carefully throughout the protracted hospital stay.[12]

On arrival at the fever hospital, patients were placed in isolation cubicles – they were not allowed to read, get out of bed, sit up or eat. Drug therapy for the treatment of typhoid fever had not yet been discovered and the only regime of treatment was to put the body into a complete rest situation and allow nature to take its course. Patients were given a small drink every two hours, one ounce of lukewarm water mixed with one ounce of milk and a salt water enema every second day. This regime was continued for six weeks when a little light food was introduced and, after eight to ten weeks, they were allowed to get up for short periods and walk outside their rooms and into the open air of the grounds. After three successive negative test results, the patients were discharged from hospital to begin the long convalescence required. On average, they lost two to three stones in weight during the disease process and were debilitated and depressed for many months following discharge.[13]

By the end of the year, the typhoid epidemic was over and the transfer of teaching arrangements to Wolverhampton took place in January 1949.

NOTES

[1] Roberts, H., student memories 1943–1948

[2] Carter, M., *Healing & Hope*, Robert Jones and Agnes Hunt Orthopaedic and District NHS Trust, 2000

[3] *The Heritage of Oswestry – The origin and development of the Robert Jones and Agnes Hunt Orthopaedic Hospital, Oswestry, 1900–1975,* Oswestry, The Robert Jones and Agnes Hunt Orthopaedic Hospital, 1975

[4] 'The Fire and After', *Orthopaedic Illustrated*, issue no. 12, p.11, winter 1971

[5] Orritt, N., student memories, 1943–1948

[6] Ibid

[7] Talbot, D., Letter to CSP Council, 5 February 1948

[8] 'The Fire and After', 1971, op. cit.

[9] Roberts, student memories, op. cit.

[10] Ibid

[11] Ibid

[12] Ibid

[13] Ibid

Chapter 8
Course Affiliation – Wolverhampton: 1949–1957

Affiliation of the Robert Jones and Agnes Hunt Orthopaedic Hospital with the Royal Hospital, Wolverhampton, was an innovative concept. The hospitals devised a course that guaranteed to qualifiers both membership of the CSP and acceptance for employment by the new NHS. As the NHS was not yet constrained by defined geographic operational parameters, there was more flexibility in the system than was apparent later, which facilitated the course development. Also, development of the Oswestry/Wolverhampton joint school of physiotherapy provided each institution with the opportunity to fulfil desires long held. Wolverhampton had for many years nurtured the ambition to establish a training course for physiotherapists, but had neither the administrative and educational expertise nor the financial resources to convert their aspirations into reality. Oswestry, on the other hand, had abundant experience and considerable expertise in the development and implementation of training courses for the ISTMS and the CSMMG, but now lacked access to particular areas of clinical experience essential for their course to transfer to the new CSP curriculum and qualification. As each unit could satisfy the other's needs, the affiliation was expected to be a success.

Initially the transfer of the school to the Royal Hospital Wolverhampton was delayed by the typhoid epidemic at the RJAH and the thirteen students scheduled to start the physiotherapy course there in September 1948 remained in quarantine at Oswestry. They were, by October, helping the hospital through the staffing crisis caused by the epidemic by nursing half-time on the wards and working the other half in the physiotherapy department. Fortunately, only one student in this set developed the disease. Also in October, a member of the physiotherapy department staff, Miss Thorpe, left Oswestry and after a quarantine period spent at her home, transferred to Wolverhampton where she started to organise the clinical education programme that students would follow on the new course.[1] This quarantine period was necessary to ensure the infection was not carried from one hospital site to the other.

The school base at the Robert Jones and Agnes Hunt Orthopaedic Hospital was closed finally for eighteen months on 4 December 1948 and arrangements were made to open at the Royal Hospital, Wolverhampton, on 1 January 1949. The four-week quarantine break allowed Dorothy Talbot and Elsa John to organise the new school teaching accommodation before students returned from their own Christmas break. The original proposal for the course was that both students and teaching staff would remain at Wolverhampton until the results of the Preliminary CSP examination were announced in June 1950. Following success in this examination, students would return to Oswestry for a further eighteen months' tuition. Any student who failed the Preliminary examination would remain in Wolverhampton until November when the resit examinations were held. These arrangements were necessary as Oswestry would no longer have the facilities or staff resources to teach subjects covered by the Preliminary examination once the transfer had been completed.[2]

By July 1949, the course was progressing satisfactorily, having overcome many of the initial teething problems, and staff worked unstintingly to ensure success of the innovative scheme. As the affiliated school was a completely new venture, formal approval by the CSP was required following careful review of all aspects of the course. This was undertaken by an inspection conducted at the school sites in February 1950.[3] Miss Summerhays and Miss Owtram, principals of Kings College Hospital and Manchester Royal Infirmary Schools of Physiotherapy respectively, represented the Chartered Society and they were requested particularly to explore the nature of the relationship between the two hospitals supporting the training school. Miss Talbot, appointed principal of the new Oswestry/Wolverhampton Physiotherapy School, had organised the course most efficiently, implementing her many decisions with skill and foresight, making full use of very limited resources. Existing staffing of the school was considered adequate for the current student numbers, but it was recognised that as additional cohorts were recruited, more teachers would be required. The situation would have been partly resolved by employment of Miss Howl, the physiotherapist scheduled to start teacher training in March 1950, but, unfortunately, she left the course after only two months in training.

The inspection team also reviewed progress on the building of the clinical and training facilities at Oswestry following the 1948 fire and were impressed by the quality of the new physiotherapy department and school under construction. They noted that, when finished, it would provide two lecture rooms, a practical classroom, gymnasium, study and changing/cloakroom for staff, but, sadly, no student changing facilities or toilet/showers for staff or students. The inspectors found the students keen and enthusiastic about their course; they treated patients with confidence and the school's examination results were satisfactory.

When applying for initial approval for the school base to be established at Wolverhampton, it had been decided to offer places to students of both sexes as there were few opportunities for young men to train for physiotherapy in Great Britain. One of the conditions of affiliation was that direct entrants to the Wolverhampton course should be offered the opportunity to train as orthopaedic nurses if they wished. It was incumbent on Oswestry, therefore, to present proposals for the accommodation of male students should this offer be accepted. In the event, only one male candidate followed the full five years' training to achieve the dual qualification and no further young men were accepted for the physiotherapy course until the 1981 intake.[4]

The inspectors commented on the excellence of the orthopaedic experience available to students at Oswestry, but also identified that, in spite of the Wolverhampton affiliation, students still did not have the opportunity to treat patients suffering from medical or neurological conditions. Miss Talbot was advised to investigate the possibility of arranging more placements in other hospitals to compensate for this deficit in the Wolverhampton experience.

Following the CSP inspection, Miss Talbot's plans for continuation of staff support of the Wolverhampton school were implemented. From March 1950, Miss John was scheduled to return to Oswestry permanently while Mr Gifford and Miss Elder (Wolverhampton employees) continued to work exclusively at the Wolverhampton base. Miss Talbot, the principal, would spend three days each week at Wolverhampton and two days at Oswestry.[5]

Before 1948, any qualified physiotherapist interested in student education could be employed in a teaching capacity in a school. However, as teachers tended to work in isolation with little peer support, it was difficult to persuade physiotherapists to leave the camaraderie of the clinical field to pursue a career in education. Schools faced permanent shortages on teaching staff establishments but often accepted the compromise situation of employment of clinical physiotherapists that enabled them to satisfy curriculum demands and enrich the student experience. Clinical staff could and did undertake course teaching, sharing their experience and expertise with students in the school while still maintaining their main clinical role in patient care.

Unfortunately, this arrangement ended with the introduction of the National Health Service as schools of physiotherapy were subsequently permitted to employ only qualified teachers, student teachers and educational gymnasts on school establishments. This imposed significant additional pressure on the schools and highlighted the severity of the crisis in teaching. After July 1948, candidates who expressed an interest in teaching now had to pursue a further arduous training course and succeed in advanced professional examinations, meaning a very high calibre of entrant was required. In spite of the high examination standard and the lack of attention paid to learning the skills required for teaching, aspiring members of this branch of the profession would not have been daunted if there had been significant rewards to be gained from the additional qualification. The reality of the situation was that teachers worked longer hours than their clinical counterparts for very little difference in salary, although they did receive an additional week in annual leave. Promotion was slow and, when it came, there was little further enhancement of salary or status.

Principals fought a constant battle trying to recruit and retain staff to maintain course teaching of an acceptable standard.

Dorothy Talbot was very active in trying to persuade suitable candidates to apply for the teacher-training course and briefed them well before they embarked on the programme. Unfortunately, two of these potential teachers failed to cope with the academic level required, withdrawing after two and four months respectively. During these early years, Jean Rogers, who qualified as a teacher in December 1956, was the only successful candidate recruited.

The relationship of the school to the hospital was also causing Dorothy Talbot many problems. Dame Agnes had started massage training as an extension of orthopaedic nursing in an attempt to satisfy the needs of patients with skeletal tuberculosis and other orthopaedic problems. The school was part of the nursing establishment and, until the end of the Second World War, teaching staff were given nursing titles – for example, Miss Dalton, the principal of the school is referred to as 'Sister Tutor' throughout the hospital's recorded minutes of meetings. The principal had no autonomy within her sphere of professional responsibility and no direct access to the hospital's decision-making body, the Hospital Management Committee (HMC). One small example of the extent of this bizarre situation was demonstrated when the Association of Orthopaedic Physiotherapists wished to hold a conference at Oswestry. On receipt of this application, the hospital's nursing subcommittee proposed that Dorothy Talbot, the principal of the school, should be given facilities to organise the meeting. However, when the recommendation was presented to the HMC, it was determined that Miss Talbot's name had been submitted in error and should be deleted, replaced by that of Miss Bell, matron of the hospital.[6] There is also evidence of lack of understanding by the HMC of the pressures on the school, biased reporting of events and considerable inflexibility in the managerial relationships which gives the inaccurate impression of the school and its potential. Its apparent loss of direction was largely due to inappropriate decision-making by experienced people who lacked the knowledge and understanding of the specific needs of physiotherapy education and who were immersed in the traditions of the hospital. These people were well intentioned and felt they were acting in the best interests of the school yet seldom, if ever, considered consulting with the principal or her staff on matters directly related to their sphere of expertise.

At Oswestry, Matron Bell had sole responsibility for physiotherapy student recruitment, one of the situations destined to produce strained relationships. As a direct result of the lack of input by the school into the selection process, some candidates with insufficient academic potential were offered places on the physiotherapy course. Their presence placed additional burdens on an already overstretched teaching staff as weaker students required more teaching input to enable them to gain professional status. The CSP urged Miss Talbot to improve the academic calibre of her students and were displeased when she appeared not to comply with their request. Owing to the idiosyncrasies of the selection process, these instructions were to no avail. In all aspects of the school's life this nursing dominance caused stress as school staff struggled to meet CSP requirements in an environment that was anchored too firmly in the past.

Matron was concerned primarily with easing the hospital's staffing situation in relation to student nurses and paid little attention to the future courses to be followed by the probationers she accepted. During the 1950s, the majority of the probationers accepted wished to pursue physiotherapy rather than general nursing once they had gained the Orthopaedic Nursing Certificate and the school was only equipped to support an annual intake of twenty students. If more students were accepted, an increase in teaching establishment would be required, but the continuing national shortage of physiotherapy teachers indicated that there was little hope of recruiting anyone to occupy the new posts created. Additional student numbers would also require significant expansion of the clinical education programme, more classroom accommodation and extra equipment, and there would be insufficient accommodation available in the Nurses' Home.

Careful preparation had preceded the affiliation with Wolverhampton; however, unforeseen events can disrupt the most meticulous planning. Typhoid had delayed the start and, exactly a month after the CSP inspection, twelve Oswestry candidates who had completed the Certificate in Orthopaedic Nursing were unable to proceed to Wolverhampton as scheduled because there were apparently no vacancies. Despite the original agreements made concerning biannual admissions, these students were obliged to start their general physiotherapy course at the RJAH and did not transfer to Wolverhampton until June.[7]

When the programme had been in operation for two years, the Hospital Management Committees decided that the hospitals should consolidate the situation by the formulation of a binding agreement to ensure continuance of the course. The agreement was to be subject to a three-year rolling contract, with twelve months' notice required for termination. This was to allow time to make alternative arrangements for the course without penalising the students already embarked on their studies.[8]

Operation of the course was proving to be a very complicated logistical exercise. Students who failed the Preliminary examination, inability to recruit a successful student teacher, additional cohorts attending the course and the distance between the two sites produced a very stressful working environment for teachers. With the overall increase in course length, staff found it impossible to teach students adequately and also supervise their practical work. There was hope in the long term for some alleviation of the staffing crisis by acceptance of Mrs Jean Rogers, an Oswestry-trained physiotherapist working at Chirk Hospital, as a student teacher. The HMC agreed to this appointment and, in April 1951, Jean took the first tentative steps towards what was to prove a long, successful career in teaching.[9]

Meanwhile the rebuilding of the physiotherapy department at Oswestry was well under way and it was decided to name the lecture rooms and classrooms after people who had made a significant contribution to the hospital's development, rather than following the previous practice of giving them numbers. The exercise practical room, the Green Room, was to be named after the Chairman of the HMC, Major Lindsay Bury, and the theory classroom, the Red Room, after the former matron, Miss Evelyn Murray.[10] The third classroom, the Blue Room, devoted mainly to the teaching of electrotherapy, was named after Avis Sankey, long-time aftercare superintendent and companion to Dame Agnes following Emily Goodford's death. In 1989, following significant upgrading of the school premises, a second theory room, the Pink Room, was created out of the south end of the Lindsay Bury Room and, following tradition, the last matron of the hospital, Miss Mary Powell, agreed to allow the room to bear her name.

On Tuesday, 11 September 1951, physiotherapy staff vacated the temporary accommodation they had occupied in Kenyon Ward since February 1948 and moved into the incomplete new physiotherapy department.[11] One of the most obvious differences between the new building and the ones it replaced was that the classrooms were no longer at ground level and, when first occupied, the floors and the treads of the stairs were still rough uncovered concrete. A design defect was the absence of toilets in the new school premises. Approximately 100 people worked continuously and studied in the school with the nearest toilet facilities on the ground floor off the south side of the main corridor, by Kenyon Ward.

Despite the dust and clamour of continuing building work, students moved into the classrooms and happily continued their studies until, one morning, they were informed the stairs were now due to be finished and would be out of use for a few days. This caused considerable consternation as these students were studying hard for the Intermediate professional examinations, a major hurdle on the route to qualification, that were due to be held a few weeks in the future. They had already suffered many setbacks during their training, including the hospital fire, the typhoid epidemic, delay in starting the course at Wolverhampton and the use of temporary study facilities when they returned to Oswestry. The final straw was to be denied access to the classrooms as they prepared for the most difficult range of examinations of their career.

Eventually, the students negotiated for a ladder to be strategically placed so that they could climb on to the roof and enter the school classrooms without using the stairs – an arrangement made for evacuation of the first storey in the event of fire. The students were quite content to use this means of access and egress and, for three weeks, both students and staff battled the elements to climb the ladder in order to reach class and changing rooms while the stairs were being covered with their terrazzo finish. Climbing a fifteen-foot ladder in a gale, wearing uniform and a cloak, which acted like a cross between a sail and a parachute, was found to be quite a challenging way to enter the upper storey of the building, but did allow the students continuity in their studies.[12]

Considering the hospital's history, it is surprising that the architects had not incorporated an effective method for evacuation of the school in an emergency. If the stairs could not be used, people in the offices and classrooms of the school were to leave the building by the French windows to access the adjacent flat roof. They were then to move across to the roof of the main corridor where a light alloy ladder was provided to give them the means to descend to ground level.[13] The hospital was, in later years, meticulous in many aspects of health and safety with compulsory student and staff attendance at regular lectures and fire drills.

Definition of the safe alternative route for evacuation of the school if the stairs were out of use was always of concern to staff but never appeared to be considered seriously by the authorities. The potential dangers of the situation were highlighted early one Friday afternoon in the 1980s when the stairs were unexpectedly out of commission for several hours. Students and staff became increasingly concerned as time dragged on and personal, social and travel arrangements were being rescheduled by the minute. The lack of toilet facilities on the upper floor contributed to the discomfort of the forty-odd staff and students trapped there. After about three hours, a student followed the hospital's instructions for emergency evacuation and, having climbed on to the flat roof, went to the point identified as the position of the ladder – but there was no ladder in place. When further assistance was requested, the message was received that nobody should go on the roof under any circumstances as it was considered too dangerous. Fortunately, hospital management responded positively to the ultimatum with which they were then presented and, within minutes, provided the required assistance for staff and students to escape from and gain access to the school during the remainder of the emergency. The school is now based at Keele University and the hospital space it once occupied is used for another purpose. Students are no longer at risk but the interested observer would, however, notice there is now a strong, permanent external spiral staircase in place should first-floor occupants of the building ever require to descend to ground level without using the normal stairs. It is only a pity that it took half a century to get round to building it.

Students are the lifeblood of any institution and they, in turn, often develop lasting friendships during their student years. This was a characteristic of all hospital schools of physiotherapy, but at Oswestry the friendships were stronger and the loyalty to their alma mater more firmly entrenched owing to the five-year contact they had enjoyed during the combined nursing/physiotherapy course. Late in 1955, the physiotherapy students decided to form an association for qualifiers from the school. Mary Powell, who had previously qualified as both an orthopaedic nurse and physiotherapist and was now an assistant matron at the hospital, was very supportive of their aspirations and encouraged them to approach the nursing subcommittee for advice on the submission of a detailed proposal.[14] The organisation, named the Old Oswestrian Physiotherapists Association (OOPA), held its first meeting on 19 May 1956 when over sixty people attended, representing many of the cohorts to have qualified from the hospital. The following year, Sir Reginald Watson-Jones lectured to more than ninety delegates attending the meeting.[15]

For nearly half a century, the organisation provided an annual opportunity for past qualifiers to revisit the hospital to renew old friendships and make contact with former colleagues. However, graduates from the Keele course did not have the same sense of Oswestry as their alma mater and recruitment since the 1994 course had been negligible, so membership levels fell. In 2002 and 2003, there were joint meetings of OOPA with the companion younger organisation, the Oswestry League of Nurses, and on 8 May 2004 the forty-ninth and last meeting of the organisation was held and was attended, as had been the first, by approximately sixty members. After considering all possible options for continuance, it was decided to disband the organisation while it was still viable and active, and to request membership of the League of Oswestry Nurses for members who wished to retain links with the hospital on a social/professional/personal basis. It was a poignant moment of regretful realism when it was accepted that the strong loyalty and identification with hospital-based professional education courses had not survived the transfer of these same courses to their current university bases.

By 1956, when the course had been in operation for six years, the Oswestry HMC was showing signs of dissatisfaction with certain aspects of the affiliation. The quality of course instruction generally was not criticised, but the committee was concerned that students now received significantly less instruction in orthopaedic physiotherapy than they had when the course was exclusively Oswestry-based. There were also major concerns about continuing low staff establishments in physiotherapy and specific staff shortages at Wolverhampton necessitating additional teaching support one day a week by Oswestry-based teachers.[16]

It was considered that four teachers and a gymnast were required for the school and a superintendent and six staff to run the department, an increase of one on the existing establishment. Unfortunately, there were only two qualified teachers in post, and Jean Rogers, due to qualify as a teacher in late 1956. The fourth post was occupied by a clinical physiotherapist.[17] The teaching situation was potentially eased in 1956 when Mrs Barbara (Bobbie) Goff was approved by the CSP for teacher training. As she was employed on a part-time basis, it was considered she would take some time to qualify. However, her family was settled in Oswestry and she was expected to remain in the area on qualification as a teacher.[18]

The Oswestry HMC continued to question the length of the period of student secondment to Wolverhampton, particularly as the hospital had never managed to provide the promised complete range of clinical experience required by students following the CSP curriculum. To compensate for some of the Wolverhampton deficits, Dorothy Talbot had organised additional placements in ante- and post-natal care at the Oswestry and District Hospital and in respiratory care at the Market Drayton chest clinic. The Oswestry HMC considered that, under these circumstances, students would now gain nothing by remaining at Wolverhampton for the full period of secondment previously agreed. They recognised that a shorter period could not be introduced immediately, as they wished to minimise the disruption of the course for direct entrants to the Wolverhampton school.

Wolverhampton Group HMC had now gained experience in course implementation and had developed a core staff with the confidence to take responsibility for operating the course independently, so it seemed to be a suitable time to consider annulment of the agreement of affiliation. After some further discussion, the agreement of affiliation was terminated and the last students to be involved in the Wolverhampton experience left the hospital on 17 May 1957.[19] Although the formal affiliation had ceased to exist, the relationship between the two schools remained cordial. For the next decade, when staffing levels permitted, Wolverhampton students attended Oswestry for one or two weeks each year to observe specialist orthopaedic physiotherapy.

Now that the logistical problems of course implementation at Wolverhampton had outweighed any advantages of affiliation, the possibility of providing the required range of clinical experience in hospitals nearer to Oswestry had to be explored. After due consideration, Miss Talbot found the Maelor and Accident Hospitals in Wrexham were of inadequate size and had insufficient equipment to support student training and she decided to enter discussions with the Royal Salop Infirmary.

Physiotherapy courses also organised additional lectures for students in specialist subjects that were expected to be outwith the expertise of the teaching staff and, for Oswestry junior students, attendance at Liverpool University was organised for anatomy demonstrations and practical physiology work prior to their entry to the CSP Preliminary examination.[20] Senior students were given courses of lectures in the treatment of medical and surgical conditions not encompassed by orthopaedics to compensate for those lost by severance of the Wolverhampton affiliation. In addition, lectures were given by physiotherapists practising in mental health, treating patients suffering from cerebral palsy and practising new massage techniques.[21]

During the 1950s, the majority of physiotherapy schools were experiencing difficulty in filling their student cohorts, whereas the courses based in London and at Oswestry had significantly more applicants than could be accommodated. The main reason for the popularity of the Oswestry course was that tuition fees were waived and accommodation was provided for all candidates who remained at the hospital to gain the physiotherapy qualification once they had completed the ONC course. This was quite a consideration in post-war Britain, as tuition fees of approximately £100/year and accommodation costs for the thirty-eight months of training made these courses too expensive for the average household to consider. CSP course entry requirements were amended in 1957 to request five O-level passes instead of four, with applicants having a wider choice of subjects from which to select. It was hoped the increased choice would have a positive influence on recruitment generally and would enable the majority of candidates to achieve academic pre-entry requirements by seventeen years of age which would enable them to start professional training at eighteen.[22]

Imminence of course changes that were to return students full-time to Oswestry led Miss Talbot to submit a proposal to the HMC that was designed to produce a higher level of coordination of student training, more effective departmental management and greater efficiency in the use of limited resources. It was proposed these plans should be reviewed after a trial period of one year. In the detail of her proposal, she demonstrated her clarity of thought and her breadth of vision once more. Against the flow of current thinking, she separated clinical and teaching responsibilities and also took account of individual personal preferences.

In September 1953, the departmental superintendent had indicated she did not wish to retain the title, and so it was proposed she, Miss Decima Hayden, be regraded as Senior Physiotherapist with responsibilities for coordination of all ward-based treatments. Mrs Tudor, a senior physiotherapist, was to be responsible for coordinating outpatient treatments with help from one assistant; the other four assistant physiotherapists who completed the clinical staff were to be in charge of two or three wards each. There was to be one male assistant physiotherapist to assist with the treatment of patients who had suffered spinal injury.

Advisor physiotherapists were qualified teachers who would give support and assistance to junior assistant physiotherapists when they first took charge of a ward. They would also be responsible for supervising the work of the students while they were gaining clinical experience. Elsa John would take responsibility for coordinating all the clinical experience gained by students away from the RJAH base and Dorothy Talbot was to coordinate the activities of the department and training school. When the proposal was presented to the nursing subcommittee, a necessary intermediary step to the HMC, there was immediate controversy. The Medical Advisory Committee, when appraised of the proposals, voiced the opinion that a hospital the size and with the reputation of the RJAH should have a superintendent physiotherapist; whereas the nursing subcommittee was prepared to allow the scheme to run for one year with the temporary elimination of the post.[23]

Eventually, the committee decided the proposal should be researched further before any decision was made. The personnel may have changed over the years, but the cumbersome decision-making processes of the hospital appeared to have been passed seamlessly from one generation to the next. Unfortunately, events took another turn as the superintendent became ill and Jean Rogers, now a qualified teacher, acted as her locum for the duration of her illness, while the other teachers shared Jean's teaching duties.[24] In view of this development, the Medical Advisory Committee felt unable to comment on the staffing arrangements proposed earlier and delayed the decision for a further six months. The HMC was, however, aware of the many staffing problems in physiotherapy and formally congratulated Miss Talbot on her approach. HMC members considered the staffing proposal Miss Talbot had already presented to the committee could be implemented effectively when Miss Hayden returned from sick leave.[25]

Notes

[1] Extracts from the minutes of the meeting of the Board of Management of the RJAH Orthopaedic Hospital, 17 October 1948

[2] Extracts from the minutes of the meeting of the Board of Management of the RJAH Orthopaedic Hospital, 18 November 1948

[3] Extracts from the minutes of the meeting of the Board of Management of the RJAH Orthopaedic Hospital, 7 April 1950

[4] Extracts from the minutes of the meeting of the Hospital Management Committee of the RJAH Orthopaedic Hospital, 27 April 1950

[5] Extracts from the report of a meeting about the physiotherapy training school held at the RJAH, 26 July 1949

[6] Extracts from the minutes of the meeting of the Hospital Management Committee of the RJAH Orthopaedic Hospital, 31 March 1955

[7] Extracts from the minutes of the meeting of the Hospital Management Committee of the RJAH Orthopaedic Hospital, 11 March 1950

[8] Extracts from the minutes of the meeting of the Hospital Management Committee of the RJAH Orthopaedic Hospital, 22 February 1951

[9] Extracts from the minutes of the meeting of the Hospital Management Committee of the RJAH Orthopaedic Hospital, 26 April 1951

[10] Extracts from the minutes of the meeting of the Hospital Management Committee of the RJAH Orthopaedic Hospital, 22 February 1951

[11] Extracts from the minutes of the meeting of the Hospital Management Committee of the RJAH Orthopaedic Hospital, 27 September 1951

[12] 'The Fire and After', *Orthopaedic Illustrated*, issue no. 12, p.11–12, winter 1971

[13] Extracts from the minutes of the meeting of the Hospital Management Committee of the RJAH Orthopaedic Hospital, 4 January 1951

[14] Extracts from the minutes of the meeting of the Hospital Management Committee of the RJAH Orthopaedic Hospital, 8 December 1955

[15] Extracts from the minutes of the Hospital Management Committee of the RJAH Orthopaedic Hospital, 28 March 1957

[16] Extracts from the minutes of the meeting of the Hospital Management Committee of the RJAH Orthopaedic Hospital, 26 July 1956

[17] Extracts from the minutes of the meeting of the Hospital Management Committee of the RJAH Orthopaedic Hospital, 28 April 1955

[18] Extracts from the minutes of the meeting of the Hospital Management Committee of the RJAH Orthopaedic Hospital, 28 April 1955

[19] Extracts from the minutes of the meeting of the Hospital Management Committee of the RJAH Orthopaedic Hospital, 31 January 1957

[20] Extracts from the minutes of the meeting of the Hospital Management Committee of the RJAH Orthopaedic Hospital, 28 February 1957

[21] Extracts from the minutes of the meeting of the Hospital Management Committee of the RJAH Orthopaedic Hospital, 29 May 1958

[22] Extracts from the minutes of the meeting of the Hospital Management Committee of the RJAH Orthopaedic Hospital, 30 May 1957

[23] Extracts from the minutes of the meeting of the Hospital Management Committee of the RJAH Orthopaedic Hospital, 26 September 1957

[24] Extracts from the minutes of the meeting of the Hospital Management Committee of the RJAH Orthopaedic Hospital, 27 February 1958

[25] Extracts from the minutes of the meeting of the Hospital Management Committee of the RJAH Orthopaedic Hospital, 27 March 1958

Chapter 9
Affiliation with the Royal Salop Infirmary: 1957–1969

On detailed evaluation, it was considered the departments at the Royal Salop Infirmary and the Copthorne Hospital would probably be able to present the range of clinical opportunity required to satisfy the CSP curriculum. It was necessary, however, to increase the physiotherapy staff at the Royal Salop infirmary by at least two full-time people to ensure the department would not be relying too heavily on the work undertaken by students as part of their course. Whereas, when the affiliation with Wolverhampton had been discussed seven years earlier, it had been determined it required four students to treat the same number of patients as one qualified member of staff would cope with, this had now been adjusted to three. It could be that over the intervening years between the two sets of discussions, the number of hours worked by students had been increased, or the inherent value of this cheap labour source was valued more highly by budget-conscious hospital management committees. Whatever the reason behind the calculation change, students made an integral and quantifiable contribution to patient care in physiotherapy departments and it was to be some years before they were to be considered supernumerary to the workforce.

The CSP arranged for the physiotherapy departments to be inspected before giving permission for the school to affiliate with the Shrewsbury Hospitals.[1] As a result of this inspection it was determined that the new liaison with Shrewsbury would be in place to start in September 1957 following some further discussions on the detail of implementation of the proposals between the Oswestry and Shrewsbury HMCs.

With minimal preparation therefore and very little fuss, students started attending the Shrewsbury departments and, after two months, favourable reports were received from the superintendent. At the Copthorne Hospital, a classroom had been provided and equipped for teaching of both practical and theoretical classes. Students travelled to Shrewsbury each day from Oswestry to gain a wider range of clinical experience, but early enthusiasm for the programme quickly palled and it was noted, over a period of time, that the daily travelling had an adverse effect on the quality of work produced. Students breakfasted at 07.00, left Oswestry at 07.45 and started on the wards and departments in Shrewsbury at 09.00. By the time they returned to Oswestry, in time for their evening meal, they were too tired to do any valid study.

Shrewsbury hospitals were able to provide only a very limited range of non-orthopaedic clinical experience and this meant the school was obliged to maintain arrangements made at the Oswestry and District Hospital and the Market Drayton chest clinic. At that time also, due to the absence of qualified physiotherapists at the Market Drayton chest clinic, students were temporarily unable to gain experience in respiratory physiotherapy until new staff appointments were made.[2] The clinical education programme was now becoming fragmented, spread over a minimum of five sites in two counties, a complicating factor for the organisers aiming for parity and acceptability of students' experience.

Due mainly to the increasing student numbers, all the negotiated clinical education bases were filled to capacity and yet were barely satisfying course requirements. As a temporary improvement, but never considered a long-term solution, Dorothy Talbot decided to establish a physiotherapy service for the treatment of elderly patients at the Morda Hospital and further placements were negotiated at the Derwen Cripples Training College. In addition to providing extra placements, this arrangement would be of advantage to patients from both locations as they would no longer be required to travel by ambulance to the orthopaedic hospital for treatment.[3]

The HMC considered that the most effective manner to deal with these many problems of the clinical education programme and the school generally was to set up a working party to report back to a future meeting of the nursing subcommittee. Dorothy

Talbot, the principal of the school, was invited to participate in the working party that was to make wide-ranging recommendations concerning the numbers of teaching staff, general practical training, classroom accommodation and equipment required by the school. Student accommodation and any other points that were considered pertinent to the school's problems were also to be included in the discussions.[4]

Another quinquennial CSP inspection was imminent and was conducted on 13 March 1959 with Miss Hawley, professional representative of the CSP, Dr Lloyd from Cardiff and Miss Evans from Guy's Hospital school of physiotherapy acting as inspectors.[5] The inspectors recommended that the school's teaching establishment should be increased by two qualified members of staff. An alternative method of calculation, as the school was considering reverting to biannual intakes, determined the increase would need to accommodate the principal and one teacher for each of the six cohorts that would be in the school at any one time. The school also needed another theoretical classroom, a changing room and a study room for students. These additional facilities were all to be allocated to the school by December 1960. Finally, the inspectors considered students' study options would be improved if the school could obtain and use dissected anatomical specimens to be kept at the hospital. This would obviate the need for students to make the long journey to the medical school at Liverpool for this essential component of the course.[6]

Minor alterations to course examinations came into force in 1957. There was a slight increase in pressure on staff as the implementation of the final examinations was increased from two to four sessions each year. Candidates who failed the final examination would still have to remain in training for an additional ten weeks prior to their second attempt to qualify. However, with the Final examination now being held in November, February, May and July, there would be less time lost prior to qualification than with the biannual examinations these new arrangements replaced.[7]

Following the award of the Royal Charter to the professional organisation in June 1920, the society had continued to seek protection for the general public from unscrupulous practitioners by statutory regulation of the practice of physiotherapy. This was introduced finally in the early 1960s after a documented campaign of fifty-five years' duration. Although now replaced by the Health Professions Council, the Council for Professions Supplementary to Medicine (CPSM) was, for forty years, the registration body for several professions including physiotherapy.[8] Acceptance of registration by the CPSM was recognition that the practitioner had undergone a period of pre-qualification instruction and, by having passed a series of professional examinations, was worthy of the title State Registered Physiotherapist. State registration has been a prerequisite of employment in the NHS since the CPSM came into being. The practice of physiotherapy is now under the statutory regulation of the Health Professions Council and, from July 2005, the titles 'Physiotherapist' and 'Physical Therapist' have been protected by HPC legislation.[9] This protection of title has not as yet been extended to cover physiotherapists in veterinary practice.

The Physiotherapists' Board of the CPSM was given the task of monitoring and reviewing CSP-approved courses and, from 1960, school inspections were carried out by the CPSM with representation by the CSP, rather than by the CSP alone.[10]

Dorothy Talbot was responsible for maintenance of both the clinical and tutorial physiotherapy services in the hospital. When, in 1960, the physiotherapist in charge of the outpatients department, Mrs Tudor, was appointed superintendent physiotherapist at the Derwen Cripples Training College, she was replaced by Joyce Bentley. Joyce, a former student of the school, had qualified in 1950 and, by December 1965, Miss Talbot, still beset by staff shortages in the school, appointed her superintendent of the physiotherapy department.

Teaching staff shortages were causing great problems, as one of their number, Diana Kidd, was terminally ill and there were, in addition, two teaching vacancies on the establishment.[11] However, staff shortages were not confined to the school as, by December 1960, partly as a result of the high proportion of student nurses opting to study physiotherapy on completion of the ONC course, there were significant shortages of orthopaedic trained nursing staff to service the wards. The Medical Advisory Committee was so concerned about the shortages of nursing staff that senior physiotherapy students were invited to work part-time on the wards during evenings and at weekends. When the proposal was put to the students, many of them agreed to help and undertook nursing duties in addition to their physiotherapy studies.[12]

Three years after the CSP inspection and four years after the establishment of the working party to address the situation, sadly no progress had been made on the accommodation issues highlighted. As there were scheduled to be six cohorts studying in the school by the end of 1962, it was considered that no more students could be admitted as the accommodation was sufficient for an annual intake, not the biannual intakes that existed.[13]

Although the HMC agreed additional classroom accommodation in the school was urgently required, they responded by establishing yet another subcommittee. The purpose of these new discussions was to explore, with the Medical Advisory Committee, the possibility of providing alternative accommodation within the hospital for the complete department.[14] This was not a very practical solution and it was then proposed that the school have use of the complete upper floor of the existing building it occupied. The pathology department, which had occupied space on the first floor since the department was rebuilt after the fire in 1948, would have to be relocated. It was situated in the second room on the right from the landing at the top of the stairs, space that was logically part of the school anyway and was later converted first into the students' common room and, later, into offices for the principal and her secretary. However, the lockable walk-in cupboard in the room was traditionally referred to as the path lab cupboard until the school vacated the premises in 1994.

The pathology laboratory was already scheduled to be relocated in the new research block, which was still under construction, and arrangements were made for it to be housed temporarily in the existing research unit.[15] That seventeen students were admitted in early October is a matter of record despite the fact the new classroom accommodation was not yet available and students still had no space in the school in which to study.

Miss Bell, matron of the hospital, retired in 1961, and Len

Hodkinson, principal nursing tutor, was appointed acting matron for twelve months. He was followed by Mary Rowlands, assistant matron and home sister, for a further period of time as a permanent appointment of matron had yet to be made. In October, after six months in this capacity, Miss Rowlands returned to her previously held position as Mary Powell had been appointed matron of the hospital. Miss Powell's qualifications for the post were exemplary. She had trained as an orthopaedic nurse and physiotherapist at Oswestry in the 1930s before continuing her career in orthopaedic nursing. During the war she had taken charge of one of the children's annexes and, later, had written the definitive textbook on orthopaedic nursing. She had served as assistant matron at Oswestry and for ten years as matron of the Wingfield Morris Orthopaedic Hospital at Oxford prior to her appointment as matron of the hospital she first joined as a staff nurse in 1936.

Communication between the hospital and the school of physiotherapy immediately improved. It had always been of great concern to the CSP and Dorothy Talbot that students entered the school without prior interview by physiotherapy staff and Mary Powell introduced radical changes to the system. Routine selection of entrants to the orthopaedic nursing/physiotherapy course was, from the time of her appointment, conducted by Mary Powell and Dorothy Talbot, representing the two components of the course to which these candidates were making a commitment.

The system worked well and a further initiative was introduced to encourage recruitment of direct entry candidates, who would be offered the opportunity to undertake orthopaedic nursing on completion of their physiotherapy studies. The proposal to reverse the two training courses arose following the transfer of student support from education authorities to the Department of Health in September 1961. As education grants for physiotherapy had been discretionary and the DOH bursaries would be mandatory, the improvement was obvious. The negative aspect of the proposal was that, although there was to be no change to the physiotherapy programme, students who had received bursaries were expected to commit themselves to two years' service in the NHS on qualification. This service requirement, following the five years' study already undertaken, meant a seven-year commitment for Oswestry students. In order to relieve this perceived hardship, it was proposed to reverse the order of the courses and encourage direct entrants to undertake the orthopaedic nursing course once they had gained MCSP. The Ministry of Health was asked to approve the proposed course in orthopaedic nursing to be followed by direct entry candidates, so that it could be counted as part of the payback NHS service required by physiotherapists who had received bursaries as students. Mr Roaf, Director of Clinical Studies, and Mr Len Hodkinson, principal nursing tutor, would join Miss Talbot for the interview of candidates for this course.[16]

Unfortunately, following a meeting of the Joint Examination Board (JEB) of the British Orthopaedic Association and the Central Council for the Care of Cripples, the JEB objected strongly to the fifteen-month course proposed prior to the award of the Orthopaedic Nursing certificate. Their main objection was that the proposed course would incorporate minimal nursing experience on the wards and they were adamant they would not allow qualification on this basis under any circumstances.

Throughout these negotiations and course modifications, students attended courses, took examinations and left for work in other hospitals on completion of their time at Oswestry. The student cohort who completed their studies in 1962 has vivid memories of the time spent in the school. All examinations were taken at a central location in Queens Square, London, and Oswestry students found it a terrifying ordeal, travelling to London and meeting with students from all the London schools in this soulless, five-storey building. They felt like country bumpkins alongside the apparently more sophisticated southern students, but the reality of the situation is that their two years' nursing experience had given them an air of confidence and made them appear more at ease than their colleagues from other schools. Many experienced physiotherapists still bear the scars of visits to Queens Square.

These former students vividly recall Bobbie Goff as a student teacher. Bobbie had two favourite sayings: 'in a nutshell' and 'take a piece of rough paper'. One day when Bobbie said 'take a piece of rough paper', all the students took out a piece of sandpaper and proceeded to sharpen their pencils on it. Bobbie was very nervous on the day of her teaching assessment, but the students who were to act as models for one of the assessed classes placed, as a good luck message, a walnut shell on her desk with the message, Postural Drainage – in a nutshell! Apparently during the class, Bobbie used the analogy of striking the base of a sauce bottle to get the sauce out to describe the removal of excess secretions from the chest. These students retained this concept throughout their working lives.

Diana Kidd made a great impression on them. She was an excellent teacher who must have taught them movement. They used to dread practical classes when all the students in the class would be sitting in a semicircle with heads bowed. Miss Kidd would announce, for example, 'Now we will have a demonstration of back extension exercises. Miss Jones you will be the model and...' She would cast her eye over the semicircle of bowed heads and when she eventually nominated the person to demonstrate the teaching of the exercises, an audible sigh of relief passed round the remainder of the group.

Elsa John taught these students massage and insisted on the removal of watches and jewellery before the class started. As students practised the various techniques on each other, she would walk around the classroom, notebook and pencil in hand, sketching the students. Unfortunately, none of these sketches survive. She is reported to have recorded faults of performance such as the 'sniff sniff technique'. Here the student, so intent on accurate performance of the particular technique, had lowered her head to such an extent that her nose was almost in contact with the model's back.

At an early stage in the course, Miss John wanted to demonstrate leg massage and of course, a model was called for. 'Who has the smoothest legs?' she asked before demonstrating her skills. Occasionally, Elsa John taught anatomy and the most significant time during her classes was spent by students struggling to copy the wonderful anatomical diagrams Elsa John, a competent artist, could produce on the chalkboard in a moment. Students with less artistic talent had little chance to reproduce the diagrams in a similar manner, but learned their anatomy thoroughly none the less. It was a pity these works of art had such a short life span as they were erased at the end of the lesson.

Dorothy Talbot taught the majority of the anatomy syllabus and, in addition to being an excellent teacher, she had an infectious enthusiasm for the subject. To encourage students to study, she always announced the proposed content of the next lesson before departing. Students remember on one occasion that she said, as she was leaving the room, 'Tomorrow we are going to study an exciting little muscle – platysma.' The majority of physiotherapists would probably be hard pressed to remember exactly the position, form and function of this muscle, but the 1959–1962 Oswestry students have no problems in this regard. Platysma is such an 'exciting little muscle' they have never forgotten it!

Students always seemed to be changing their clothes. For clinical practice and theory classes in the school, they wore white overalls and white caps. Gym was taught by Miss Kempster, the educational gymnast employed by the school, and for her classes and all other practical sessions, blue aertex shirts, grey shorts and unflattering grey gym knickers were worn.[17]

A significant part of their clinical experience was gained at the orthopaedic hospital but, in addition, they attended Market Drayton, NSRI, RSI, Copthorne Hospital and finally the Oswestry and District and Morda Hospitals nearer home. Elsa John supervised their clinical work at Morda and students remember when her little VW beetle was seen approaching the hospital, they would become frantically active, dashing up and down the staircases and corridors of the rambling building, keeping out of her way. At lunchtime, they gathered at the entrance for a lift back to the hospital and were really surprised she had not been able to find them when they were working on patients.

The other clear memory is the chore of tidying the departments before finishing for the day. Slings, ropes and pulleys were hung neatly ready for use next session, SWD and UVL rooms were tidied with electrodes stacked, gym mats were piled one on top of the other and, worst of all, the wax room was thoroughly cleaned and the used wax boiled and cleaned for reuse. On Fridays the plinth covers and pillowcases were changed and all surfaces cleaned and polished.

These were the students who were also among those offered the opportunity to work on the wards to alleviate the staffing crisis in nursing and this was a very popular option as they were paid Staff Nurse rates for their times on duty. A pleasant end to their studies that lightened the spirits of staff at this stressful time occurred in early December 1962, when the CSP examination results were published. Despite all the traumatic events of the past year, the thirteen students who entered the Final examination in November all passed at the first attempt.[18] It appears from the Hospital Management Committee minutes that 100 per cent success in the Final examination occurred in two consecutive years. It was therefore either this group or the set immediately below them who celebrated the publication of their examination results by being loaded into ambulances and touring the lanes and byways around the hospital with horns and sirens blaring, lights flashing and streamers flying in recognition of their achievement.

The school's staffing problems were compounded by the fact that Diana Kidd had died in August 1962 after her long illness. She was greatly missed by both staff and students. Another student teacher was recruited and it was hoped she would eventually be a replacement for Diana,[19] but she left the course after only two months' training.

By this time, Jean Rogers was a competent, confident teacher with five years' experience. She made a successful application to join the CSP panel of examiners in September 1961.[20] This was very useful to the school as the CSP operated a national examination system. An examiner had the opportunity to review the quality of work produced by students from other schools, identify strengths and weaknesses of the system and improve the syllabus of teaching in his/her own school if areas of specific weakness were discovered. As interschool communications were still infrequent and of limited value, this was an effective way to exchange ideas.

Dorothy Talbot had over the years successfully recruited Jean

Rogers and Bobbie Goff, who qualified as teachers in December 1956 and 1960. The staffing situation looked as if it would improve slightly when Madge Graveling, who had trained at the hospital between 1945 and 1950, applied and was accepted for the emergency teacher training course introduced by the CSP in 1962. This course was developed in response to the continuing desperate national shortage of teachers and was only to run for one cohort. It involved two months' training in London followed by four months' teaching practice in a recognised training school and was designed specifically for senior and experienced physiotherapists in an attempt to ease the crisis in teaching.[21] Applicants now learned more about techniques of teaching and examining and less about advanced anatomy and physiology than in the previous course.

The course started on 17 October 1961. Students returned to their training schools in January 1962 and took the qualifying examination at the end of April. Madge Graveling was expected to be successful in gaining the Teaching Diploma and had made a commitment to stay on the school staff for at least a year after qualification. On completion of her contracted year she asked to be relieved from her post to return to clinical work. As the other student teacher taking the earlier long course had also left, the school lost a further two full-time staff and had received no applications for the vacant positions. Miss Joan Cash, remembered for her pioneering books on physiotherapeutic management of patients with surgical and medical conditions, had, by that time, retired from full-time teaching, but was persuaded to help out the school for two days a week.[22]

The hospital was by now very concerned about the problems of the staffing and establishment of the school and constituted a subcommittee in 1963 to discuss the matter. This committee had Mr G.K. Rose, Mr R. Roaf, Mr T. Lythgoe, Mrs Langshaw Rowland, Miss M. Powell (matron), Miss D. Talbot (principal) and Mr P.J. Challinor (secretary to the HMC) as members.[23]

The Chartered Society was also well aware of the extreme staffing problems experienced by the majority of schools and developed another course for potential teachers that was hoped to ease recruitment to this beleaguered branch of the profession.

This course, offering the qualification of Diploma of Teaching in Physiotherapy (Dip TP), was to be of seventeen months' duration, starting with two months' attendance at the Polytechnic of North London (PNL), allowing students to learn many educational aspects of teaching and examining on adult, professionally based courses. After ten months at the hosting training school, a further four weeks' attendance at the Polytechnic was required before the student teacher's classroom abilities were assessed by a senior physiotherapy teacher and an educational psychologist. The Ministry of Health had provided funds and made provision for thirty-five student teachers to be trained each year, but, although the target was reached with the first cohort, the following year recruitment dropped to sixteen physiotherapists, not all of whom completed the course. The numbers achieved in the first year of operation were never to be repeated.[24]

Miss Winifred (Wyn) Cannell, an experienced physiotherapist who had recently returned from Kenya, was appointed to start as a student teacher at Oswestry on 1 September 1964, five months prior to enrolment on the new Diploma of Teaching course, which started in February 1965.[25]

The school continued for several more months with Dorothy Talbot, Elsa John, Jean Rogers, Bobbie Goff and Greta Anderson employed full-time, Joan Cash helping out and Wyn Cannell attending as part of her teacher-training course. Ann Savin, another qualified teacher recently returned from a post held in South Africa, eased the situation when she accepted a position on the teaching staff on 23 May 1966, a month before Wyn was to have her final assessment.[26]

In June 1964, the first school inspection conducted by the statutory body, the CPSM, with the professional body (the CSP) in attendance, was undertaken by Dr Dobny, Miss Elphick, principal of St Thomas' Hospital school of physiotherapy and Miss Sybil Evans, principal of Guy's Hospital school of physiotherapy. The inspectors visited classes, clinical areas in the North Staffordshire Royal Infirmary, the Shrewsbury Hospital Group, Oswestry and District Hospital and the Derwen Cripples Training College. As Miss Talbot explained, the school had now reached the full six sets of students resulting from the build-up of the biannual admissions started in 1962, and accommodation needs were pressing. Students were in urgent need of study space in the school, as, during term time, when the classrooms were in full use, they were obliged to sit in their cloakroom to study. The school library stock was held in a cupboard in the corridor, so was not able to be used fully.

The inspectors' recommendations were quite helpful to the school as they addressed the problems with which Miss Talbot and her staff had been battling for some time. Ironically, the inspectors recommended and the HMC accepted that the establishment should be increased by one and that teachers in post should attend more post-registration courses for updating of professional knowledge. Their main concerns, however, related to the level of accommodation provision for students. The HMC referred the provision of an additional library/study room, tutorial room, student common room and staff changing room to the building subcommittee for action.[27]

As can be imagined, there was considerable annoyance expressed by the HMC when they were apprised of the extent of the CPSM's demands for additional accommodation in the school. They recalled the transfer of the pathology laboratory to another location in 1962 and implied that the hospital had been put to this great inconvenience in order that the space vacated could be used as an additional lecture room. Miss Talbot had, however, used the space as a study/library for the students. The building subcommittee had also proposed that the board room in the medical records block could be used for study purposes when not required for meetings, but as the desks would have to be removed prior to each meeting, this proposal was impractical. The board room was more suited to be a lecture room, but again it was not a practical proposition owing to the necessity for the removal of the furniture prior to each board meeting.[28] This was an effective impasse and the committee decided that no further action should be taken on the matter of finding additional accommodation for the school.[29]

The MOH had approved a new syllabus for training that was due to start with all students commencing courses in 1965. The dates of admission and the examinations were altered slightly, but the length of training remained unchanged. The new syllabus required sixty lectures in surgical and medical subjects by members of the medical profession and twenty-four demonstrations in anatomy and physiology in medical school. Lectures in psychology and practical courses in gymnastics and remedial games were still required.[30]

Dorothy Talbot was very concerned to find a permanent solution to the many problems surrounding the range and quality of clinical experience available to her students. Association with Wolverhampton and Shrewsbury had enriched the student experience somewhat, but had not solved the underlying problems of the range and quality of clinical experience required to satisfy the CSP curriculum. Rather than continuing to develop more and more small satellite units, she aimed to make a final affiliation to enable the clinical education programme to be concentrated on major hospital sites.

Her enquiries led to Stoke-on-Trent and a preliminary meeting was arranged for 27 February 1963 between the group secretary and officers of the Stoke HMC and representatives from Oswestry. It was agreed that the secretary, Mr P.J. Challinor, Miss D.F. Talbot, principal of the school of physiotherapy, Miss M. Powell, matron of the hospital, and Mr R. Roaf, Director of Clinical Studies and Research, would represent the RJAH. Following this meeting, a report was to be prepared and submitted to the nursing subcommittee at Oswestry.[31]

A second meeting was arranged for 6 June 1963 and it was hoped that, after this had taken place, a joint memorandum would be prepared laying out the principles for the proposed agreement of affiliation.[32] The memorandum was prepared and forwarded to the Stoke HMC for consideration and approval before presentation to the Oswestry HMC in September.[33] Matters proceeded as predicted and, on receiving the memorandum following its approval by the Stoke-on-Trent HMC, the Oswestry HMC determined that closer integration with Stoke-on-Trent should be introduced immediately and eventual affiliation of the Physiotherapy training between Oswestry and Stoke-on-Trent should be considered.[34] Further discussion was recommended between Miss Powell, Miss Talbot and Mr Challinor before the scheme was implemented.[35] These discussions took place and Miss Talbot submitted a report to the nursing subcommittee that unfortunately is not available and no record of its contents have been found.[36] No further action seems to have been taken on this proposal although, at the CPSM/CSP inspection in June 1964, it was recommended that efforts be made to secure affiliation of the school with the NSRI. The inspectors considered that closer liaison with the Stoke-on-Trent hospitals would provide a wider range of clinical experience for students, but there would be staffing implications. They hoped that, when finally implemented, the affiliation would provide proper safeguards for the Oswestry school, a cryptic and possibly perceptive comment to make on such a brief contact.

When the inspection report was received by the HMC, it was reported that discussions with the CPSM/CSP inspectors had deviated from the detail of the proposed development with Stoke-on-Trent to which the HMC had agreed. Miss Talbot was asked therefore to resubmit the proposals she had outlined to the inspectors, to the MAC and to another subcommittee consisting of Mrs Langshaw Rowland, Mr McSweeney and Dr Johnson for further consideration.[37] All negotiations and discussion of the topic appear to have come to a halt at this stage and no further activity was reported to the HMC. Students were, however, being seconded to the North Staffordshire Royal Infirmary to gain experience in the treatment of patients admitted to the neurology, neurosurgery and thoracic surgery units.

By 1967, Dorothy Talbot was quite exhausted. She had used her abilities and intellect for twenty years trying to keep the course running at the hospital and had had more than her fair share of problems. During her tenure of post, she had coped with the hospital fire, typhoid epidemic, introduction of the NHS, affiliations of the course with Wolverhampton and Shrewsbury and had managed to retain her enthusiasm. She continued to try to further discussion on the proposed affiliation with Stoke-on-Trent, but, as Stoke was unlikely to become a medical teaching centre in the foreseeable future, no further discussions were to be held and the proposed affiliation was dropped down the hospital's list of priorities.[38]

Lack of interest in the school's welfare, lack of autonomy in her area of professional responsibility and the constant irritations caused by the relationship of the school to the hospital's management structure encouraged her to consider retirement. At this point Dorothy Talbot informed the CSP and the HMC that she had tendered her resignation and would surrender her post in February 1968, three months after Elsa John would have retired. The Education Committee of the CSP expressed their regret that she should now be considering retirement as her valuable experience as principal would be lost to the school at a vital time. The HMC made no comment.

She was very interested in a new form of treatment, Maitland's mobilisations, and wished to travel to Australia to meet with Geoff Maitland and learn the skills of his approach. In June 1967 she carried out a final duty on behalf of the CSP by assessing a student teacher at the Bradford Hospitals School of Physiotherapy. For the student teacher, Marian Hilton, it was a day that determined the course of her future life as Miss Talbot, unable to give her the results of the assessment, offered her a post on the teaching staff at Oswestry. Marian decided to accept the offer for September 1968 and was destined to arrive in Oswestry, fourteen years after she had made her first unsuccessful application for a place on the April 1955 ONC course.

The CPSM/CSP inspection of the school was carried out on 17 and 18 April 1967, when the inspectors again commented on the superior abilities in handling and management of patients demonstrated by students who had previously gained the Orthopaedic Nursing Certificate. They were, however, very concerned about the seven-year commitment made by these students to the profession and noted that almost a third of those accepted on the course failed to qualify. It was thought the combined training would not continue unless radical alterations were made to the nursing component in order to retain the competitiveness of the school in relation to other physiotherapy courses.

Significant changes in the structure of the orthopaedic nursing course had already been presented to the Orthopaedic Nursing Council for consideration, and on this submission were found to be acceptable. The new proposal was that students would enter the course at seventeen, spend one year orthopaedic nursing followed by three years' physiotherapy training. An optional six months of concentrated orthopaedic nursing training would follow, while the candidates were paid on the basic physiotherapy salary scale and they would then be able to take the examinations for the award of the Orthopaedic Nursing Certificate. Those who did not wish to take the additional training would become qualified physiotherapists and would be issued with a statement confirming their year of orthopaedic nursing.

The CPSM report continued with the warning that, despite the excellence of the orthopaedic experience, arrangements made for clinical education in the treatment of patients with non-orthopaedic conditions were considered to be unsatisfactory. During the visit the inspectors had met with representatives of the North Staffordshire Royal Infirmary Stoke-on-Trent and were impressed by the apparently genuine desire on the part of the North Staffordshire Management Committee to play a part in providing facilities to extend the experience of the Oswestry students.[39] Sadly, following the inspection, the report delivered the ultimatum that unless the school made a definite affiliation with a general hospital, the course would no longer be acceptable for state registration purposes. The deadline for submission of these proposals was to be the end of the year.

A positive benefit of the 1967 inspection was stimulation of the hospital's interest in the school. Mr Slee, a senior orthopaedic surgeon, and Dr Ward, a consultant rheumatologist, had been delegated specifically to show interest in the work of the department.[40] Dr Ward was particularly conscientious and for many years gave unstinting support to the school and the principal.

Dorothy Talbot retired, as she had planned, in February 1968, and as a tribute at her leaving party students performed sketches highlighting the strengths and characteristics of individual staff members. Although now many of the comments would be considered politically incorrect, all contributions were greatly appreciated and enjoyed on the occasion they were presented. The sketch performed by the finalists is clearly remembered by Rachel Jordan, who was then in the first six months of the physiotherapy course. Bobbie Goff, by now an experienced teacher and an expert in neurology, was particularly interested in the normal neurological development of children. Finalist students dressed in nappies and little else performed to music an excellent demonstration of child development over the first two years of life. The sketch was a roaring success and Rachel admits she cannot remember any of the other contributions, as they were all overshadowed by the finalists' presentation.

NOTES

[1] Extracts from the minutes of the RJAH Orthopaedic Hospital Management Committee meeting, 27 September 1956

[2] Extracts from the minutes of the RJAH Orthopaedic Hospital Management Committee meting, 28 November 1957

[3] Extracts from the minutes of the RJAH Orthopaedic Hospital Management Committee meeting, 18 December 1958

[4] Extracts from the minutes of the RJAH Orthopaedic Hospital Management Committee meeting, 26 June 1958

[5] Extracts from the minutes of the RJAH Orthopaedic Hospital Management Committee meeting, 26 March 1959

[6] Extracts from the minutes of the RJAH Orthopaedic Hospital Management Committee meeting, 30 April 1959

[7] Extracts from the minutes of the RJAH Orthopaedic Hospital Management Committee meeting, 31 May 1955

[8] Tidswell, M., 'Physiotherapy: A True Profession?', unpublished MA dissertation, 1991

[9] Health Professions order 2001, Statutory Instrument 2002 no. 254

[10] Tidswell, 'Physiotherapy: A True Profession?', op. cit.

[11] Extracts from the minutes of the RJAH Orthopaedic Hospital Management Committee meeting, 24 November 1960

[12] Extracts from the minutes of the RJAH Orthopaedic Hospital Management Committee meeting, 30 March 1961

[13] Extracts from the minutes of the RJAH Orthopaedic Hospital Management Committee meeting, 25 January 1962

[14] Extracts from the minutes of the RJAH Orthopaedic Hospital Management Committee meeting, 26 July 1962

[15] Extracts from the minutes of the RJAH Orthopaedic Hospital Management Committee meeting, 18 October 1962

[16] Extracts from the minutes of the RJAH Orthopaedic Hospital Management Committee meeting, 30 November 1961

[17] Student memories 1959–1962

[18] Extracts from the minutes of the RJAH Orthopaedic Hospital Management Committee meeting, 27 December 1962

[19] Extracts from the minutes of the RJAH Orthopaedic Hospital Management Committee meeting, 29 November 1962

[20] Extracts from the minutes of the RJAH Orthopaedic Hospital Management Committee meeting, 26 October 1961

[21] Extracts from papers attached to the minutes of the RJAH Orthopaedic Hospital Management Committee meeting, 28 September 1961

[22] Extracts from the minutes of the RJAH Orthopaedic Hospital Management Committee meeting, 25 April 1963

[23] Extracts from the minutes of the RJAH Orthopaedic Hospital Management Committee meeting, 30 May 1963

[24] Extracts from the minutes of the RJAH Orthopaedic Hospital Management Committee meeting, 30 December 1965

[25] Extracts from the minutes of the RJAH Orthopaedic Hospital Management Committee meeting, 30 July 1964

[26] Extracts from the minutes of the RJAH Orthopaedic Hospital Management Committee meeting, 29 June 1966

[27] Extracts from the minutes of the RJAH Orthopaedic Hospital Management Committee meeting, 29 October 1964

[28] Extracts from the minutes of the RJAH Orthopaedic Hospital Management Committee meeting, 28 January 1965

[29] Extracts from the minutes of the RJAH Orthopaedic Hospital Management Committee meeting, 25 March 1965

[30] Extracts from the minutes of the RJAH Orthopaedic Hospital Management Committee meeting, 31 December 1964

[31] Extracts from the minutes of the RJAH Orthopaedic Hospital Management Committee meeting, 28 February 1963

[32] Extracts from the minutes of the RJAH Orthopaedic Hospital Management Committee meeting, 30 May 1963

[33] Extracts from the minutes of the RJAH Orthopaedic Hospital Management Committee meeting, 19 June 1963

[34] Extracts from the minutes of the RJAH Orthopaedic Hospital Management Committee meeting, 26 September 1963

[35] Extract from the minutes of the RJAH Orthopaedic Hospital Management Committee meeting, 31 October 1963

[36] Extracts from the minutes of the RJAH Orthopaedic Hospital Management Committee meeting, 30 January 1964

[37] Extracts from the minutes of the RJAH Orthopaedic Hospital Management Committee meeting, 29 October 1964

[38] Extract from the minutes of the Education Committee of the Chartered Society of Physiotherapy, 3 March 1967

[39] Extracts from the report of the visit by the Physiotherapists' Board of the CPSM, 17–18 April 1967

[40] Extracts from the minutes of the RJAH Orthopaedic Hospital Management Committee, 29 October 1964

Chapter 10
The Oswestry and North Staffordshire School of Physiotherapy: 1969–1974

Miss Margaret (Greta) Anderson, a member of the teaching staff, replaced Dorothy Talbot as principal in February 1968. Jean Rogers was appointed assistant principal and Bobbie Goff and Wyn Cannell occupied teaching posts. Ann Savin had left the school in December 1967, leaving two vacant posts on the establishment. Marian Hilton came to the school from the Bradford Hospitals School of Physiotherapy in September 1968.

Immediately following confirmation of her appointment, Miss Anderson notified the CSP that Oswestry had decided to revert to an annual student intake from October 1968.[1] She also invited Miss Orme, principal of the London Hospital School of Physiotherapy, to visit Oswestry on behalf of the CSP on 3 March 1969 to review progress on the affiliation with Stoke-on-Trent and to advise on the means to an effective conclusion of negotiations.

It appeared that the Stoke HMC was still willing for the affiliation to take place. Although the hospital authorities had assured Dorothy Talbot some months earlier that the idea of a closer association with the NSRI was not a matter of immediate practical politics, the hospital was now actively searching for appropriate teaching space and residential accommodation for the school and students. A teaching post had been created for Stoke-on-Trent, but no applications had been received, which meant the new facility would have to be serviced by existing Oswestry teaching staff, replicating the situation that had existed following affiliation with Wolverhampton twenty years earlier.

Teaching accommodation was eventually found in the Harrison Hut, a temporary wooden structure, the front part of which was used for the treatment of patients with neurological problems. Students and staff had to time their arrivals and departures carefully so that treatments were not interrupted.

Prior to signing the agreements of affiliation, the hospital management committees developed the mechanisms necessary to determine appropriate funding, management and lines of communication for the school. It was quite a complicated situation as all costs associated with the establishment of the school and its future operation were to be shared by the two separate hospital management committees at a time when cross-boundary flow of personnel and resources was not usual practice in the NHS. It was important to establish a workable structure without having the benefit of reference to procedural guidelines drawn up by other institutions attempting similar arrangements.

The level of commitment by the two management committees to the project is exemplified by the manner in which these individual problems were addressed and successfully resolved. It was determined there would be a school committee which would, through its membership, report directly to each HMC. This committee, the Education Committee of the Oswestry and North Staffordshire School of Physiotherapy, was cumbersome but well meaning and steered the school through the early days of affiliation with an unexpected confidence and competence. Once established, it convened a subcommittee, the Academic Review Board, with the brief to assist the principal to deal appropriately with students who had failed to satisfy the school or CSP examiners. This subcommittee had the authority and power to terminate the course for persistent failures and give encouragement and support to those who were trying but had difficulty with the intellectual level required to succeed on the course and examinations. The committee supported the principal, confirmed her recommendations and supported the predetermined draconian action with students who were persistently failing at every level of examination.

Representing Oswestry on the Education Committee were Dr Ward and Mr Slee, a consultant rheumatologist and an orthopaedic surgeon respectively, who were, following recommendations made by an earlier inspection team, already taking an official interest in the school's activities. Mrs Gwynne, a lay member of the HMC, Miss Anderson and Mrs Rogers, the principal and assistant principal of the school, Miss Powell, matron of the RJAH and two administrators, Mr D. Cruttenden and Mr W. Colbert, completed the Oswestry team. Stoke-on-Trent had a similar representation with Mrs Robinson, lay member of the HMC, Mr Crowe and Mr Walker, consultant surgeons at the NSRI, Miss Birchenough and Mrs Harrison, superintendent physiotherapists from the North Staffordshire Royal Infirmary and City General Hospital and finally, Mr Lowndes, an administrator.[2] As people moved to other posts or retired from the committee, they were replaced by the new incumbents to the posts vacated which meant there was a dynamic element to the group while maintaining a stable core of its membership.

A new school badge was designed that incorporated elements from the original Oswestry badge offered to students on qualification with the Staffordshire knot and the potter's wheel. The design was finalised in time for it to be awarded to the students who qualified in November 1970. The badge with which they were awarded had a base of white metal and cost a mere 14/6 to make. It would have been more in style with the rhetoric and declared enthusiasm for the course if the committee had agreed the same design in sterling silver although the cost would have mounted to £3/6/6d. per badge. A badge made from silver indicates the donors are proud of their product whereas one in white metal confirms that the institution has taken the cheapest option available and in so doing, the mark of achievement given to students at the end of an arduous course is somewhat devalued.[3] The first time the badge was presented was in July 1971, when twelve students – nine first entrants and three retakes – all passed the examination. Mrs Gwynne, the Chairman of the Education Committee, made a congratulatory speech and presented the badges in the gymnasium at the RJAH with the students and staff in attendance.[4]

It was decided that meetings of the Education Committee would be held quarterly, the venue alternating between Oswestry and Stoke-on-Trent, and the chairmanship was to be taken by the lay representatives on the committee. Mrs Pat Gwynne was elected the first chairman, a post she held for about fifteen years. She was conscientious, enthusiastic and very sincere. At the first meeting of the committee, final plans for the affiliation were made and the official start date of the new school was determined to be 15 May 1969. Although the new teaching post based at Stoke-on-Trent had been advertised, Miss Anderson had received no applications and proposed to service the venture from Oswestry if an appointment could not be made in time. To encourage applications, it was proposed to regrade the post as assistant principal before resubmission of the advertisement. Although the MOH recommended that there should be only one assistant principal to a school, the precedent for appointment of an assistant principal at each of the established bases of this school was accepted. The ONSSP then became the only physiotherapy school in the country to have two assistant principal posts although, sadly, one of them was unoccupied for most of the time it was in existence.

The arrangement was for students to remain at Stoke-on-Trent for a total of twelve months over the second and third years of the course. While there they would be seconded to wards and departments at the NSRI and CGH where experience in general medicine, general surgery, obstetrics and gynaecology, ENT surgery, dermatology, thoracic surgery, neurosurgery and neurology would be gained. Residential accommodation was to be organised for students and for the teachers from Oswestry who would service the school pending an appropriate appointment being made to the Stoke-on-Trent post.[5] Greta Anderson spent the first month after affiliation at Stoke-on-Trent and, on her return to Oswestry, the other teachers each spent a month in turn, when they worked Mondays and Fridays at Oswestry, and Tuesdays, Wednesdays and Thursdays at Stoke-on-Trent. It was arranged that medical staff would lecture to the students on Friday afternoons when teaching staff had returned to Oswestry, but how well these lectures were attended is not known.

Teachers also had clinical duties to fulfil at Oswestry as they were appointed physiotherapists in charge of wards at the RJAH. It was a little bizarre, for the month of their secondment to Stoke, to review patients on Monday with the senior student, who was then left in charge to report the patients' progress to the teacher on her return from Stoke-on-Trent on Friday. Most students were excellent, mature and competent in manner and practice, accepting the responsibilities they were given and reporting back effectively at the end of the week. Occasionally, the arrangement was an unmitigated disaster; it all depended on the quality of the student in charge.

There was, at the time of the affiliation, stark contrast between the levels of provision in the main Stoke-on-Trent hospitals. North Staffordshire Royal Infirmary was a voluntary hospital prior to the introduction of the NHS. It occupies a commanding position at the top of a hill and looks down on the Central Outpatients and City General Hospital. This slight elevation gave it a psychological boost seldom vocalised, but evident from the attitudes of the staff and the work that had devolved to each hospital. The City General Hospital was at a disadvantage owing to its origins and also the fact it was built on lower ground than the voluntary hospital. It was difficult initially to dispel the workhouse image and the hospital was obliged to retain the original buildings for decades, adapting them with variable success for effective use in a technology-led medical environment. The end result of these perceived discrepancies was that City General Hospital developed specialisms less dependent on technological support that could be accommodated in the rabbit warren of buildings that was the hospital's legacy. North Staffordshire Royal Infirmary developed the high-profile surgical expertise that could be more readily accommodated in buildings that required little alteration.

The physiotherapy department at City General Hospital was a listed building. It had been built as a Victorian workhouse with small, interlinked rooms, narrow corridors and many tortuous flights of stairs in inappropriate places. There was little that could be done to make it a viable rehabilitation unit that could satisfy patient needs in the late twentieth century, and staff and students worked under extreme difficulties. Over the last three decades, the situation has changed dramatically as modern ward blocks have gradually replaced the original Victorian structures. The new rehabilitation unit, built in the second half of the 1990s, is a testament to City General Hospital's continuing commitment to improving the standards of care for patients in the area. With each new development, the morale of staff employed by the hospital has been seen to improve and the hospital is now developing many high-technology-dependent specialisms.

Stoke-on-Trent's industrial history of mining and pottery had produced a high level of atmospheric pollution and, when combined with a dusty working environment, the result was that many older patients suffered extensively from silicosis, chronic bronchitis, emphysema and many other problems resulting from their environment and lifestyle. At City General Hospital students gained an experience in the treatment of medical chest conditions that was unrivalled throughout the country. There was also a large, newly built maternity hospital, offering extensive obstetric and gynaecological experience. The remainder of the hospital was filled with general surgery cases, care of the elderly and had several medical wards occupied in equal proportions by patients who had suffered strokes or had succumbed to their chest problems. The North Staffordshire Royal Infirmary had for some time provided students with experience in thoracic and neurosurgery and now offered, additionally, intensive care, treatment of burns, a renal unit, neurology and excellent experience in a wide variety of outpatient treatments.

There were marked differences between the hospitals in all areas of activity including the quality of their nurses' home accommodation. Senior students were awarded rooms at the NSRI and had few complaints; however, the standard of accommodation offered to students by City General Hospital was appalling. The nurses' home was downtrodden, ill-furnished and poorly furbished with an atmosphere reminiscent of a neglected institution of a bygone era. It was an incredibly awful environment for the students and, for many, marred enjoyment of the quality of the clinical experience they were receiving. The stark contrast between the open aspects of Oswestry and the clutter of redbrick buildings that formed City General Hospital was the subject of comment by many of the first students to attend this new secondment. Whereas, in reports to official meetings, all students were described as happy, well settled and enjoying their new experiences, for the junior students resident at City General Hospital, their experience was largely negative. Some hated the hospital to such an extent they considered leaving the course or seeking transfer to another school to complete their studies. Many vowed they would never return to Stoke once they qualified and have been true to their word.

The Harrison Hut, the first teaching venue for the school, was a wooden building tucked away out of sight on the NSRI site. It was difficult to find, but after a few days, homing instincts prevailed and most students and staff were able to locate it without too many wrong turns on the way. Once there – provided patients were not being treated in the front portion of the building – entry could be gained to a pleasant overheated classroom behind the treatment area. Desks were in place to accommodate theoretical teaching, but practical subjects were, of necessity, taught in the physiotherapy departments of the two hospitals, during the lunch break or after patients had completed their day's work. This was not a satisfactory arrangement for students or staff, particularly if they were to return to Oswestry or beyond after they had finished teaching.

Second- and third-year students attended Stoke-on-Trent at the same time for part of the year, an interesting situation for the logistics of teaching, with one member of staff in attendance and one room in which teaching activities could be pursued. As each group was scheduled for three hours' teaching daily, even if it could be organised, the visiting teacher could not cope with six hours' teaching, student tutorials and/or counselling, clinical supervision and school administration on the one-day-a-week visit, and compromises had to be made. Students also had to get used to seeing only one member of staff for the complete month and then adjusting to a different one. Syllabus teaching tended to be uncoordinated and a little disorganised owing to the frequent changes of personnel and the limitations imposed by the arrangement of the Harrison Hut. Students could also have criticised the low level of clinical supervision on the wards, but, for the most part, they made no audible complaints and sat out their time waiting impatiently for their return to Oswestry.

By December 1969, as there had been continuing lack of

success in the recruitment of an assistant principal for Stoke-on-Trent, Greta Anderson decided that second-year students would not be seconded to Stoke until a teaching appointment had been made. Instead, they would attend the Shrewsbury hospitals to gain the experience missed by this course realignment and would therefore continue to be resident at Oswestry for the time this experience was being gained.

This solved the major problems of the level of student accommodation offered by City General Hospital, but detracted from the benefits of the quality of the clinical experience offered by the affiliation that was not working to its full capacity. Yet again, it was teaching staff shortages and the inability to recruit to the Stoke-on-Trent post that triggered the students' return to the Shrewsbury hospitals where a more limited range of experience was available. Third-year students would continue to be seconded to Stoke-on-Trent as arranged and a teacher would travel from Oswestry to provide them with one full day's teaching each week.

Finally an application was received for the Stoke-on-Trent position and Mrs Chanmugan, a qualified physiotherapy teacher, was offered the post[6] and took up her appointment on 11 May 1970. She was responsible for an exacting teaching programme for the Preliminary and Finalist students and also supervised the clinical work of second-year students in the physiotherapy department and on surgical and medical wards at City General Hospital. Once she had started work at Stoke, the school's Education Committee recognised the excessiveness of her workload and the establishment was increased by one teaching post.[7] This teaching post did not attract a single application throughout its existence and Oswestry-based staff continued to service the Stoke-on-Trent base to ease Mrs Chanmugan's burden. Wyn Cannell, who had remained on the teaching staff at Oswestry after qualifying as a teacher, tendered her resignation and left in May to take up a post in Uganda. There was, however, a net gain in teaching staff numbers as in September 1971, Ralph Kay came to the school from Northern Ireland. Continuing staff shortages, particularly at Stoke-on-Trent, caused many concerns; in addition, Marian Tidswell applied for and was granted maternity leave that was anticipated to last for four months, ending in March 1972.

Mrs Chanmugan did not stay for long and resigned from post leaving Stoke-on-Trent on 20 July 1972 to take up employment at the Fucha Institute of Rehabilitation in Tokyo. As, following a round of advertisement, there were no applications received for either of the posts at Stoke-on-Trent, full teaching cover at that school base reverted to the previous arrangements where staff from Oswestry were seconded to Stoke-on-Trent in an attempt to keep the course running.[8] The main problem with this arrangement was the continuing desperate shortages of teaching staff throughout the school and the additional burdens imposed by the necessity of providing service to the two school sites. These shortages were compounded by the fact that Marian Tidswell had still not returned to duty and there remained only four teachers in the school available to take on the additional work. It was arranged that Greta Anderson would partner Ralph Kay and Jean Rogers would partner Bobbie Goff. Each pair would undertake to travel to Stoke for a period of four to six weeks, one member of the visiting team travelling on Mondays and Fridays, the other on Tuesdays and Wednesdays.[9]

As there appeared to be no prospect of recruiting qualified teaching staff to Stoke-on-Trent, two proposals were submitted to the Education Committee. The first concerned the appointment of a clinical supervisor to undertake student supervision, relieving teachers of this responsibility. The other proposal concerned an approach to the Department of Health and Social Security (DHSS) to determine if it was possible to pay an additional allowance to teaching staff to compensate for the many excess hours they were working in order to service the Stoke-on-Trent base.[10]

The staffing situation was eased slightly when Marian Tidswell was well enough to resume part-time teaching duties in September 1972. She returned to work four days a week and, in late September, heard she had been elected as a CSP Council Member in Section 'A', the section representing teachers of physiotherapy. This was the first time that an Oswestry staff member had been elected to Council. Council members were expected to attend approximately eight meetings a year, so initially the hospital was not disadvantaged as the meetings Marian attended could be accommodated on the days she was not scheduled to work. Also, a student teacher at Oswestry, Susan Rhodes, completed the Diploma course in March 1973, but sadly did not remain at the school once she had qualified; she is believed to have left the profession altogether to pursue an alternative career. Wyn Cannell was on home leave during the summer of 1972 when the political situation in Uganda deteriorated significantly. She was advised by the Foreign Office not to return to her post in Kampala as her safety could not be guaranteed. As Wyn had bought a house and made a home in the area it was not difficult to persuade her to apply for the assistant principal post in Stoke-on-Trent.[11]

Equipment, library books and teaching aids were urgently required for the Stoke-on-Trent section of the school and the NSRI initiated an expenditure that would satisfy the most urgent needs of the school. Unfortunately, at the same meeting, it was reported that extensions to the radiotherapy department at the NSRI required the building of a wall across and through the classroom of the Harrison Hut, significantly reducing its overall size and rendering it unusable during the course of the building work.[12] Alternative accommodation was offered at the Limes, an administration building; however, the rooms allocated were very cramped and totally inadequate for teaching purposes as they could accommodate a maximum of six students when there were at least ten who needed to occupy the space. Equipment required for use in practical classes was stored in an inaccessible storeroom and was therefore unusable.[13] Miss Anderson was very concerned that the academic and practical needs of the students could not be met within the new accommodation and urged the NSRI to find more suitable rooms for the school. After some hard negotiation, additional space in the Limes was allocated but although better, it remained totally inadequate for the teaching of practical subjects or for the numbers of students requiring theoretical teaching.

There were many unfulfilled promises made by the Stoke HMC and the school was obliged to continue in these unsatisfactory conditions for more than a decade before being allocated more appropriate accommodation. The HMC had their own problems as the Birmingham Regional Health Board had promised to build a combined education centre for radiographers, physiotherapists and occupational therapists on the Stoke-on-Trent hospital site. This promise was dangled in front of the relevant schools for a number of years, but the building never came to pass. In the meantime, the schools of radiography and physiotherapy continued to occupy 'temporary' accommodation seldom fit for purpose and they struggled to maintain curriculum teaching in these adverse conditions.

It is ironical that often when there are many overwhelming problems, something happens to lighten the atmosphere. In this year of stress and gloom, the CSP awarded the Manley Memorial Prize to an Oswestry student, Penny Holden, who had qualified in November 1971. The prize was awarded annually to the student who had gained the highest marks in the Preliminary, Intermediate and Final examinations set by the CSP.[14] It was the first time the prize had been awarded to an Oswestry student and the Education Committee was fulsome in its congratulations. OOPA was also thrilled and at the Annual General Meeting of the organisation that year, Penny was awarded life membership.

There was significant increased pressure on Nurses' Home accommodation at Oswestry as students found it easier to have staff residency accommodation on their return from Stoke-on-Trent than to rent privately. The Education Committee determined, however, that rooms should be allocated initially to students starting training and that, after August 1972, second- and third-year students should find accommodation outside the hospital.[15] Following an application to the Birmingham RHB, it was anticipated that financial assistance would be provided for the building of additional residential accommodation at Oswestry. Two residential blocks were expected to be ready for occupation during the 1974/1975 financial year.

When the school reverted to an annual October intake of students, it was primarily to relieve the pressures on teaching staff as it was easier to teach three sets of students than the six produced by biannual admissions. Another consequence of the reduction in student numbers was that there were now significantly fewer students treating patients, and clinical staff numbers had to be increased.

By 1972, the combined orthopaedic nursing/physiotherapy course had virtually ended. Of the twenty-seven students accepted for the October 1972 entry, only five had preliminary nursing experience. Four had taken the year of preliminary training with the option of completing the ONC on qualification as a physiotherapist; the fifth would have completed her ONC studies prior to entering physiotherapy.[16]

The Harrison Hut was again under threat and, this time, hospital policy prevailed. The radiology department expanded further and completely obliterated the students' accommodation. Students had already lost use of part of the Hut on an earlier expansion of this department and had only been allowed limited access to the restricted space remaining in 1972. On their return, they had shared what remained of their room with occupational therapists.[17]

The school base at Oswestry demonstrated very clearly the problems of running a school without the benefit of a budget that was ring-fenced, particularly in the low level of equipment provision. By 1967, after almost twenty years of operation within the NHS, they had been able to purchase only one overhead projector for use by five teachers in four classrooms. This was used mainly by Bobbie Goff to illustrate her movement, physiology and pathology classes. She had, in common with the rest of the teachers, a very heavy teaching schedule and enjoyed the challenge of the new technology. As Bobbie would probably have five or six classes a day, it did not leave the projector unused for much of the time.

A manually operated slide projector had been offered by and gratefully received from the school of nursing when their projector was being replaced. The majority of the school's electrical and movement equipment and an anatomical model of the torso with detachable organs had either survived the fire in 1948 or had been bought to replace articles lost in the conflagration. Library books were sparse and many of the texts were out of date and had been superseded by later editions. The Lindsay Bury and Avis Sankey rooms were used primarily for teaching movement and electrotherapy, but also doubled as additional theory rooms. As there were no desks, students rested their files on the thirty-year-old examination couches, sat on low exercise stools and made the best of the inadequate conditions. The store of crutches and other walking aids that were used to teach the students crutch walking had been examined by the hospital and found to be unsafe for use by patients and, rather than being discarded, they were sent to the school. Students and teaching staff were obviously considered expendable by the hospital management.

These examples of poor teaching aid provision challenged students to find solutions to their learning requirements, and one student from Set 33 had difficulty remembering the detail of the course of peripheral nerves from their exit from the vertebral foramina. She approached Miss Anderson for permission to tape wire to one of the school skeletons, to outline the courses of the nerves in question. Slowly and laboriously, over a period of weeks, she taped pieces of wire, each following the pathway of an individual nerve from its exit at spinal level and following its detailed route to its extremity, down one side of the skeleton. She learned her anatomy and discovered that other people were using her 'learning aid' as she was asked by a fellow student if she would hurry to reach the femoral nerve, a nerve causing the student in question some problems. Mrs Rogers was also known to use this particular skeleton to teach anatomy to the year behind.[18]

School studies were augmented by visits to the Liverpool Medical School for teaching on prosecuted specimens. Students were impressed by the anatomy demonstrator who, without fail, at the end of the teaching session would say to the specimen, 'Thank you for sharing with us.' He did this even if he was using only an arm or a leg; the deepest respect was shown to the specimen that overcame the awful smell of formaldehyde and reminded students this was once a complete person.[19]

These students, being resident on site, used to practise massage in the evenings in the Lindsay Bury Room (movement classroom). One evening, there was a queue outside the door – a small bat was fluttering around inside the room and other students were concerned about entry. It fell to the student who had taped wire on to the skeleton to brave the bat, catch it and render the room 'safe' for the scheduled massage practice.[20]

At that time the school was organised on a formal basis. Students and staff wore uniform all the time they were in the school or on the wards. For ward work and theory classes, white overalls were worn with the obligatory brown or black laced shoes while for practical classes and gym students wore blue aertex shirts and gym pants under grey shorts. With this uniform, white ankle socks and plimsolls were worn. Students changed from one uniform to the other several times a day in the corridor that ran down the side of the Lindsay Bury Room that gave them easy access to movement classes. This formality in dress was carried over to the classroom as all students and staff continued to address each other by title and surname in all their dealings in classroom or clinical situations. The corridor leading to the Avis Sankey Room (electrotherapy room) was lined with approximately forty book lockers, about half the number required for each student to have a personal locker.

In anticipation of major changes in NHS management due to be implemented in April 1974, the Chartered Society published the first paper giving guidance for the clinical training of students. The first sentence must have struck a blow to many departments throughout the country and certainly the School Education Committee read it with a certain amount of gloom. The sentence read: 'It should be recognised and acknowledged by hospital staff at all levels that students attend hospital for training, not just to provide a source of labour.' The guidelines continued with an outline of the professional, educational, ethical and legal framework required to support the students' clinical education programme adequately.[21] If the Education Committee had paid due attention to these guidelines and slowly implemented the proposals outlined by the document, many of the problems the school faced over the next decade could and would have been avoided. Predictably, they made the comment that the document was of interest and then promptly forgot about it.

In March 1973 the Chartered Society of Physiotherapy put forward initial proposals for a complete review of the examination system. The existing triad of Preliminary, Intermediate and Final examinations had been in operation since 1948 and had become very jaded. Also, the pass rate at first entry to the examinations had dropped to a mere fifty to sixty per cent and, with the syllabus becoming more overcrowded each year, complete revision was required to ensure the objectives of the Society and the needs of the profession continued to be met.[22]

Significant changes in the CSP course and examination system were due to be implemented from the 1974 October intake. The course was to be reduced in length from the three years, two months to two years, nine months, in an attempt to realign it more in the style of academic years. Students who entered the course in October would take the first professional examinations the following June, consisting of papers and a structured practical examination in anatomy and physiology. During the second and third years the course would alternate clinical learning with classroom activities. The second year would end with an internal assessment. The final examination was scheduled for June of the third year of the course. There would be two papers for candidates to answer on the theory underlying the practice of physiotherapeutic procedures and a practical examination. It was in the conduct of the practical that the most change was noted as, for the first time in history, physiotherapy candidates were to examine patients. Models were to be replaced by patients examined by the candidate who would then plan an appropriate treatment programme based on the findings at examination and possibly would be asked to demonstrate aspects of this treatment. The final examination was to be held at the school with an external physiotherapist and internal medical examiners judging student performance.

Many of the hospital's doctors were initially so concerned for the well-being of their patients that they were reluctant to allow them to be involved in this new style of examination. They thought that students, under the stress of examination conditions, might do some irreparable harm to their patients, although, at all other times, they had made no complaints when the students had treated patients with only minimal supervision from qualified staff. The patients, on the other hand, thoroughly enjoyed the experience and many of their early performances were worthy of Oscar nominations. Without exception they took proprietorial interest in the result obtained by 'their' student and were quite perspicacious in their observations of the examination conduct and performance.

The medical examiners at Oswestry were at first pleasantly surprised by the practical competence demonstrated by the students and the depth and breadth of the candidates' knowledge. They took their responsibilities seriously and examined the candidates appropriately and the school was very grateful for the sympathetic support it received from the consultant orthopaedic surgeons and rheumatologists in the area. If students were unsuccessful in either of the June examinations, it was proposed they would resit in September. A second failure required the candidate to wait until the next June before another attempt could be made.

At Stoke-on-Trent, there were still problems with accommodation, equipment and books required by the school. A Kromayer lamp had been requested for teaching purposes only and was placed on the list of requests for physiotherapy equipment. Several months later it was determined that the Kromayer lamp was manufactured in Germany and could not be obtained. However, if the school wished students to gain experience in the use of this particular type of lamp, they would have to utilise existing equipment in the physiotherapy departments of the hospitals where students were seconded, provided patients were not attending for treatment.[23] By 1974 the purchase of the Kromayer lamp for the school had not been completed and students were dodging patients and using the lamps at City General Hospital and North Staffs Royal Infirmary. It was not a satisfactory situation and, without the cooperation of the physiotherapy departments concerned, students would not have been able to practise these treatments. There was to be another CPSM/CSP inspection of the school between 19 and 21 June 1974.[24]

Greta Anderson retired on 31 October 1974. Her six-year tenure of the principal's post had been dramatic and meaningful to the school's development. She had been appointed to post when the school was perched uncomfortably on the horns of a dilemma; it would be forced to close or, alternatively, make permanent arrangements with a large general hospital to ensure an adequate programme of clinical experience for the students. She had managed to finalise the arrangements for the formation of the Oswestry and North Staffordshire School of Physiotherapy and nurtured the school through the difficult early years of affiliation. The perennial problems of poor living conditions, inappropriate teaching accommodation and the minimal occupancy of the three teaching posts at Stoke all contributed to a considerable increase in the workloads that she and her staff endured to try to make a success of the venture. She had accepted this challenging post at an age when most people were thinking of retirement. However, with her devotion to duty, tidy mind, rigid self-discipline, well developed organising capabilities and the Oswestry capacity for working through what would appear to others an impossible situation, she carefully steered the school through its difficult years of initial joint management.

The staffing position continued to give great concern as, following Wyn Cannell's appointment to the post of principal in succession to Greta Anderson, the three teaching posts at Stoke-on-Trent were now vacant. Although some interest had been expressed in the clinical supervisor post, there had been absolutely no interest expressed in the two teaching posts. Teaching staff from Oswestry continued to service the Stoke-on-Trent school as best they were able in addition to their Oswestry-based teaching schedules. The only solution the committee was able to propose was that it might prove easier to recruit teaching staff to the major site of the school and proposed that there should be an increase in the Oswestry establishment. With the clinical supervisor posts at Stoke-on-Trent doubled now with one for each major hospital site, it was hoped that the quality and quantity of effective clinical supervision would improve and that the incumbents of the posts, when appointed, would be happy with their roles.[25]

NOTES

[1] Extracts from the minutes of the CSP Education Committee meeting, 21 August 1968

[2] Extracts from the minutes of the ONSSP Education Subcommittee meeting, 11 March 1969

[3] Extracts from the minutes of the ONSSP Education Committee meeting, 9 December 1970

[4] Extracts from the minutes of the ONSSP Education Committee meeting, 7 July 1971

[5] Extracts from the minutes of the ONSSP Education Subcommittee meeting, 11 June 1969

[6] Extracts from the minutes of the ONSSP Education Committee meeting, 25 February 1970

[7] Extracts from the minutes of the ONSSP Education Committee meeting, 7 July 1971

[8] Extracts from the minutes of the ONSSP Education Committee meeting, 7 June 1972

[9] Ibid

[10] Extracts from the minutes of the ONSSP Education Committee meeting, 6 September 1972

[11] Extracts from the minutes of the ONSSP Education Committee meeting, 7 July 1971

[12] Extracts from the minutes of the ONSSP Education Committee meeting, 23 March 1971

[13] Extracts from the minutes of the ONSSP Education Committee meeting, 7 July 1971

[14] Extracts from the minutes of the ONSSP Education Committee meeting, 7 June 1972

[15] Extracts from the minutes of the ONSSP Education Committee meeting, 1 March 1972

[16] Ibid

[17] Extracts from the minutes of the ONSSP Education Committee meeting, 4 April 1973

[18] Anon – Set 33 (1970–1974)

[19] Ibid

[20] Ibid

[21] CSP, *Clinical Training of Students at Schools of Physiotherapy*, 6 April 1973

[22] CSP, *Revision of arrangements for the final examination of the CSP*, 2 March 1973

[23] Extracts from the minutes of the ONSSP Education Committee meeting, 12 July 1973

[24] Extracts from the minutes of the ONSSP Education Committee meeting, 12 June 1974

[25] Extracts from the minutes of the ONSSP Education Committee meeting, 15 October 1974

Chapter 11
The Oswestry and North Staffordshire School of Physiotherapy: 1974–1981

Wyn Cannell was appointed principal of the school on Greta Anderson's retirement. She was an excellent teacher and dedicated clinician and was, until her appointment, assistant principal at the Stoke-on-Trent branch of the school. She approached her new role with energy and enthusiasm, but in addition to the normal anticipated problems encountered by a new principal in post she had to contend with others, the significance of which were not anticipated fully at the time of her appointment. She was appointed when the management of change was becoming as important an issue for principals as the efficient implementation of existing courses, and few were prepared adequately for this realignment of responsibilities. Wyn had to come to terms with major reorganisation of the NHS, establishment of a totally new pre-registration course and the consequences of the implementation of recommendations contained in the Halsbury Report.[1] These three major factors marred her tenure of the post.

Initially the NHS was characterised by medical and administrative dominance in a bureaucratic framework and, from the mid 1950s, the introduction of technical and specialist managerial staff challenged and, in some cases, undermined these traditional hierarchies and relationships. Over the next decade, piecemeal reorganisation of occupations within the service occurred, encouraging managerial attitudes among senior practitioners prior to the first major reorganisation of the NHS. This was implemented in 1974 with realignment of administrative units to produce larger, more cost-effective multidisciplinary management systems. The fourteen Regional Health Authorities (RHAs) created covered virtually unchanged geographical areas from the original RHBs and were then divided into ninety Area Health

Authorities (AHAs) that matched county council and metropolitan districts. Lines of accountability were considered very important to the efficient functioning of the new system. Authorities delegated functions to multidisciplinary teams of officers as well as to individual chief officers who formed the teams. However, the formal structure of these reforms greatly extended the lines of communication and slowed decision-making.[2]

Effectively, the 1974 reorganisation introduced another tier of management between regions and hospitals. Area Health Authorities were relatively autonomous units, responsible for the management of all resources and activities within their boundaries, and were accountable to a parent Regional Health Authority. Salop Area Health Authority was, for ease of management of the wide geographical area, also divided into sectors. The Robert Jones and Agnes Hunt Orthopaedic Hospital, the site of the main base of the school, was the largest hospital of the northern sector of Salop Area Health Authority (SAHA). By contrast, the subsidiary section of the school based at the Limes was located in the North Staffordshire Area Health Authority (NSAHA).

The CPSM, concerned about the position of schools of physiotherapy following the reorganisation, proposed that principals should arrange to be personally and directly accountable to the new Area Health Authorities.[3] The Registrar of the CPSM considered this was necessary as, owing to the financial arrangements for the support of physiotherapy education in the NHS, hospital boards of management had no means of identifying the monies allocated centrally to support this activity from within their overall budget allocations as the money to run schools, although still centrally determined, was not ring-fenced. It formed part of the common financial pool, ensuring physiotherapy educational demands were in constant competition with patient needs. These monies were frequently used to support other areas of responsibility within general hospital budgets, leaving the majority of schools significantly underfunded.

The administration of the school was now very complicated, with extended lines of communication in not one, but two Health Authorities. The problems were compounded by the fact that the main site at Oswestry was based in a 'sector', one step removed from the location of the subsidiary site in an 'area'. This made effective communication even more difficult. Education Committee members had previously discussed their role and possible position following reorganisation, but had not anticipated that the school would have different levels of accountability in the two Health Authorities. They were unsure as to how they could continue effective management of the school under these new circumstances.[4]

In Shropshire, the newly appointed administrator to the northern sector, Jeff Silk, acted as Secretary to the Education Committee and was very supportive of the school throughout his tenure of post. However, the usual pattern of activity was that, following extensive negotiation for the school's needs in both Health Authorities, Wyn discovered all too often that the school Education Committee did not support her requests. From the outset, the committee proved reluctant to take responsibility for even basic support of the school and frequently ignored published statutory guidelines for appropriate accommodation provision and course changes. There were always more pressing patient needs to swallow the limited NSAHA and SAHA budgets.

The course of training followed by schools of physiotherapy had been established in 1947 and was now jaded, no longer preparing UK physiotherapists adequately for their future professional lives. Advancements in knowledge, a clearer identification of the role of the physiotherapist and the development of rehabilitation as a scientific discipline had encouraged the CSP to update its curriculum and devise a more appropriate pre-registration course. In addition to the 'normal' problems a new principal would expect to encounter, Wyn was appointed to post within months of the introduction of this course and no one could have predicted the degree of upheaval this change would have on staff and students alike. The existing course provided an excellent practical training, with little attention to education in areas other than those subjects delineated by the curriculum of study, whereas the new course addressed education in parallel with training.

CSP had recognised that specific knowledge, on which the

previous curriculum had been based, quickly became outdated and the context in which it was applied rapidly changed. The approach of the revised syllabus was to emphasise underlying intellectual, scientific and technological principles rather than maintaining the relatively narrow specialist professional knowledge of the previous course. This demonstrated significant educational progression by the CSP, but required the design of a completely new curriculum and the learning of different techniques required by the new examination formats.

The new course mounted examinations at the end of the first and third years only, with practical skills being tested by a flexible continuing assessment system to be undertaken during the first two and a half years. The existing course held eight scheduled written and practical examinations to be completed each calendar year. During the first year of implementation of the new course, there was hardly a time when the school was not involved in preparation for, or support after, student examinations and, regrettably, the results were not always viewed with the sensitivity the students deserved.

In planning the new course, the CSP had attempted to align physiotherapy education with the timing and format of courses in the higher education sector, although there was at that time little possibility of transfer of the majority of schools to the preferred environment. The overall course length was reduced from three years, two months to two years, nine months (three academic years), with syllabus modifications to accommodate the change. The Part 1 examination was comparable with the foundation level of degree courses, taken at the end of the first year, with Part 2 equated with the standard of degree examinations occurring towards the end of the course.

The established pattern of essay-style answers to questions and practical demonstrations of techniques or knowledge was now to be interspersed with other examination formats designed to test the whole range of student ability. Teachers had already constructed a bank of multiple choice questions (MCQ) on anatomy and physiology for the CSP; however, the amount of work expended on this exercise was totally disproportionate to the value of the result. The MCQ paper initially accounted for only twenty per cent of the mark awarded to the Part 1 examination and was later reduced to ten per cent before being abandoned altogether. The other examination components, two short essay answer papers on anatomy and physiology and the demonstration of practical anatomy, were each awarded forty per cent of the total. When the MCQs were discontinued, the short answer papers contributed sixty per cent of the marks for the examination.

Part 2 candidates made a detailed study of a predetermined topic prior to sitting an open book examination to answer a question related to the topic they had studied. They were expected to analyse, evaluate, synthesise and select information that was not purely factually based. The examination demonstrated significant educational progression but had significant resource implications as students required access to many published research papers relating to the topics chosen each year. The second part of this paper, taken as a separate examination, required responses in an essay form that was familiar to staff and a further paper requested short essay answers to the ten questions posed. Each paper – Paper 1A, Paper 1B and Paper 2 – contributed twenty per cent to the final result. The examination was completed by the assessment of a patient and planning of treatment in front of two examiners, one of whom was likely to be a specialist/consultant in the hospital housing the school, the other a physiotherapist.

Several of the consultant staff from Stoke-on-Trent and Oswestry responded to the call for medical examiners to support the new examination system, although some expressed concern that students were to be assessed using real patients. When advised the examination was to resemble an over-supervised controlled section of the existing clinical education programme and that no actual treatment was to be implemented, they were reassured. Among those recruited initially were the consultant rheumatologists, Dr Ward and Dr Hothersall, a consultant physician, Dr Hart, and an orthopaedic consultant, Brian O'Connor. Brian O'Connor was appointed a CSP examiner at about the same time as he was appointed to the first Robert Jones Chair of Orthopaedics in the University of Birmingham.[5] As it required all the energies of the total teaching staff and the support of many clinicians to organise the patient assessment examinations, they were always held at Oswestry, never at Stoke-on-Trent.

The final component of the new course was the assessment of the clinical skills of physiotherapy using the Continuous Assessment Record Book (CARB). Seventy-five per cent of the listed techniques were to be assessed successfully during the first two and a half years of the course as a prerequisite to entry to the qualifying examination. These assessments were conducted in both clinical and educational settings, supposedly without disruption of the student's routine, but in reality they developed into multiple mini-tests. Barbara Shotton, principal of the Bristol School of Physiotherapy and the CARB Assessor for the Oswestry course, commented on her first visit to the school that she was most impressed by the manner in which teaching and clinical staff were cooperating to achieve the very highest possible standard of student performance.[6]

As aforementioned, Wyn faced many problems while principal and it was an unfortunate irony that the third major event to mar her enjoyment of the position was the publication of a report, long-awaited, that was hoped to remedy many of the ills of existing pay structures. The Whitley Council had been established with the introduction of the NHS to negotiate salaries and working conditions for the majority of professional staff groups, but, over the years, it had fallen into disrepute owing to the level of Treasury and DHSS control exercised. Staff had become increasingly dissatisfied with a cumbersome system that had no established criteria for determining pay rises other than the dispersal of pre-allocated amounts from the Treasury; and with no access to negotiation, arbitration or enquiry, a culture of low pay and poor working conditions had developed. Some groups – doctors and dentists, for example – had pay review bodies reporting annually to government, but others such as nurses and physiotherapists had no such arrangement. Also, as physiotherapists were members of the PT'A' Whitley Council that represented eight diverse occupations, a major flaw in the 'negotiation' situation was that awards were made to all, on a 'take it or leave it' basis, with no consideration given to the individual differences of the member professions.[7]

The first independent pay review of the professions supplementary to medicine, under the chairmanship of Lord Halsbury, published its report late in 1974.[8] Major pay awards were recommended for all staff ranging from twenty-five to eighty-five per cent, with the lowest award by many percentage points recommended for qualified teaching staff of the training schools. When enhanced by overtime, on-call payments and additional annual leave allocation, physiotherapy clinical staff almost doubled their pre-Halsbury salaries, whereas, by comparison, teachers had gained an increase in salary of approximately a quarter with no change to their leave allowance. Prior to Halsbury, teachers' salary scales had equated with those of the second highest grade of superintendent and had now been effectively reduced to the level of a Senior 1. The final anomaly was that within the PT'A' Whitley Council, physiotherapy schools alone were required to employ only qualified teachers or student teachers on their staffs. In the other professions covered by the PT'A' Whitley Council, teaching did not require additional training and clinicians/teachers were a common feature of school establishments.

Physiotherapy teachers identified that they had lost consideration for the numerous hours expended preparing for their teaching and examining activities. These had previously been recognised by the salary level and the additional week of annual leave allowance. As all staff now received the same annual leave allocation and teachers' salary relativities had been radically altered, all previous perceived recognition was lost. At the same time, teachers within the five English schools of physiotherapy based in polytechnics, but still funded by the NHS, had benefited from the major pay awards recommended by the Houghton Committee.[9] This committee had investigated the pay and conditions of academic staff in centres of higher education and their report had been published within days of Halsbury. The awards to physiotherapy teachers/lecturers in the two reports bore no comparison and the NHS was openly supporting two different salary scales and conditions of service for a group of staff performing the same range of duties.

Senior clinical physiotherapists had traditionally been

recruited to teaching, bringing experience, knowledge and wisdom to their new roles. They undertook a relatively arduous additional course and on achieving qualification, remained on virtually the same salary throughout their teaching careers. As a result of the Halsbury recommendations, the reward for this additional effort would be a substantial drop in salary, a significant consideration for any person with family responsibilities.

Morale plummeted in NHS-based physiotherapy schools. Figures collated by the CSP for the years 1974 and 1975 showed a dramatic increase in the number of teachers lost to NHS-based schools compared with earlier years and, worse, noted that applications for the teacher training course had fallen by fifty per cent.[10]

The award had been recommended for the eight PT'A' professions and as only a small section of one had been selectively adversely affected, it was accepted. There was, however, a need to restore the confidence of physiotherapy teachers before the NHS-based physiotherapy schools collapsed and this reached a successful conclusion four years later. It was a campaign that stimulated questions, debate and agreement in government and required acceptance by the Whitley Council that the original recommendation adversely affected physiotherapy alone. The council was unable to pursue an individual problem affecting a single member profession but had advised CSP that the other groups covered by the council would not object or interfere with attempts to rectify the anomaly.

The Minister of Health, David Ennals, finally admitted that the physiotherapy profession had proved its case and agreed that unacceptable anomalies had arisen as a result of implementation of the recommendations. On receipt of this information, there was muted jubilation only, as the government had introduced a period of pay restraint.[11] Teachers were pleasantly surprised therefore to find in April 1978, approximately four years after the initial award had been made, that the pre-Halsbury teaching/clinical differentials in salary levels were restored. It was anticipated the steady erosion of teaching staff from NHS schools would then cease and there was, as predicted, an immediate improvement in student teacher recruitment.[12] The Clegg

Report[13] had now been published and although it referred to the need to retain the parity between teaching and service grade salaries, the recommendations stated otherwise. For the second time, a major report altered the balance between the two sections of the physiotherapy profession, giving lower awards to teachers, reducing the pay scale from nine points to five and increasing their designated working week from thirty-six to thirty-seven and a half hours. This last point was purely academic as teaching staff were recognised as working far longer than the designated hours.[14] Fortunately, the report's recommendations with regard to physiotherapy teaching staff were almost immediately overturned.

With Wyn's appointment to the principal's post, all teachers were employed by SAHA and all the vacancies were at Stoke-on-Trent. In the past, the NSAHA-based posts had attracted little support, only being occupied for approximately three out of the seven years of their existence, and it was unlikely that recruitment could be successful in the post-Halsbury environment. The school was now in an extremely vulnerable position with only the five posts based at Oswestry occupied out of an establishment of eight. If a single teacher were to leave, the school would cease to be viable. Fortunately, no one resigned from the Oswestry staff and the school actually gained an additional teacher when Pat Wood decided to return to full-time teaching. She had been working as a teacher/supervisor at the Norfolk and Norwich Hospital and joined the staff in February 1976.[15]

Beris Jones, a senior experienced clinical physiotherapist specialising in the treatment of patients with neurological problems, was appointed clinical supervisor at the North Staffs Royal Infirmary in mid 1975. Prior to taking up the post, Beris spent an induction week at Oswestry and it was arranged she would attend the main school base one day each month to help relieve the isolation of her employment. With these visits and regular contact with the Oswestry teaching staff on both sites, it was hoped she would more readily identify her contribution to the students' learning experiences.[16] Oswestry teaching staff resumed daily travel to Stoke-on-Trent to cover essential theory and practical work. Ralph Kay and Wyn Cannell arranged to work a full day each week, when they would undertake some clinical supervision in addition to classroom activities. Jean Rogers and Marian Tidswell went for a half day only, for course teaching.

The Halsbury Report was published during the final academic year before implementation of the new course, and, although staff were keen to work as a team to devise the new curriculum, Wyn declined their offers. She determined she should take full responsibility for the new course, partly due to her position as principal and partly because she was devastated by the paucity of the Halsbury award made to the staff. She had benefited from an acceptable eighty-five per cent increase in salary and refused to accept the staff's offers to take on additional responsibilities when their award had been so derisory.

This was an unfortunate decision as no one involved in teaching at that time had experienced such radical change in the pre-registration course and staff recognised it was too great a task for one person to undertake alone. Unfortunately Wyn had also totally misjudged the level of dedication of her staff who would not allow personal disappointment to interfere with their responsibilities to the school and students. With five experienced teachers involved in planning the new course, the CPSM's comments in 1981 may have been unchanged, but teachers would have shared the responsibility. In the event, Wyn accepted sole responsibility for the course preparation and everyone was very distressed to learn the external evaluation of her efforts. The visitors commented on the lack of a coherent course plan, poor integration of the academic and practical elements of the course, and priority being given to the provision of a clinical service rather than meeting the educational needs of the students.[17] They commented further that as the allocation of teaching was subject to change and substitution with frequent modification of planned timetables, it was difficult for staff and students to plan their work or study effectively.

The Education Committee supported an application for an additional teaching post for the Oswestry base of the school to ease the almost intolerable burden being carried by teaching staff,[18] but although the AMTs approved the appointment in principle, there was no funding available to support the post. All bids for staff increases had been frozen pending an announcement by the DHSS concerning the amount of the financial allocations to be made to AHAs to offset the Halsbury pay award. When this money was made available it was hoped the funding of an additional teacher post would be approved.[19]

The school's staffing situation eased with the appointment of Lieutenant J.A. (Tony) Fowler to the assistant principal's post at Stoke-on-Trent in January 1978 on his retirement from naval service. His previous post had been principal of the Royal Naval School of Physiotherapy, Haslar.[20] Tony stayed until 1980 when he was appointed principal of the Liverpool School of Physiotherapy.[21] Some time later, in September 1979, Ralph Kay reduced his hours from full-time to four days a week.[22]

Bobbie Goff, now a very experienced teacher, had established her reputation as a national expert in the management of neurological dysfunction and had run many weekend courses, lectured to conferences and written journal articles. During 1974, she organised a course at the RJAH on behalf of the CSP on the assessment of spasticity and perceptual defects. Teaching staff contributed short talks or practical demonstrations to the sixty or so course attendees representing the wide range of professions involved in rehabilitation. Although the majority of delegates came from different parts of the UK, there were also participants from Australia, Canada and the USA. Bobbie was now consolidating her international standing. In October 1974 she presented a weekend course to qualified physiotherapists in Holland on Rood techniques; she was invited to Capetown University for a three-month lecture secondment in 1976, and in the early 1980s led a month-long course in Portugal. A member of the clinical staff, Cath Rose, also lectured on the programme in Portugal. In recognition of her contribution to and teaching of neurology, Bobbie was awarded Fellowship of the CSP in 1988. This is the highest honour the professional body can bestow on a member.[23]

Staff and students traditionally supported several voluntary activities within the hospital, but during the 1970s the time commitment required to pursue these activities eventually interfered with course operation and a significant level of tension developed. Most students at that time were resident in the hospital and were available throughout the year to push beds and wheelchairs from the wards to the Concert Hall for film shows, concerts or church services. They also assisted at the spinal injuries unit's sports weekends, provided a refreshment service for hospital visitors on Saturdays and helped with weekend riding classes for the disabled in Glyn Ceiriog. In 1977, first-year students undertook a sponsored reading of their textbook, *Gray's Anatomy*, which raised a substantial sum of money for the spinal injuries unit at the hospital. The reading was reported by Radio Stoke and the *Shropshire Star* and, subsequently, the editor of *Gray's Anatomy* included their efforts in the centenary history of the book.

Students provided the main entertainment at the hospital fête for three years in succession. The first year, 1979, they developed a cancan routine that was performed energetically and surprisingly competently to a most appreciative audience, following a late cancellation of the prearranged entertainment. After two more years of providing the main entertainment, students requested they should cease this particular activity as the hospital fête invariably coincided with the CSP examination period. The 1981 CPSM inspection report commented that the current level of voluntary activity should be reduced and student participation in hospital activities should in future be on a truly voluntary basis.[24]

Oswestry was gaining national prominence through student activities as members of the National Organisation for Physiotherapy Students (NAPS) and later as part of the physiotherapy section of the National Union for Students (NUS). They organised social events and held biannual conferences, several of which were held at Oswestry. The first one took place in 1976, but the most memorable one was in 1979. It was planned for 16 to 18 March; however, one of the speakers fell ill a few days before she was due to deliver a paper and Jean Rogers agreed to present the paper in her place. March often presents challenges for travellers and this year was no exception. About lunchtime on the Friday snow began to fall and, before long, a blizzard was in full swing. Jean left work early in the hope that the road to Glyn Ceiriog would still be accessible. Before she left, she handed over the paper to Marian, who lived in Oswestry and considered that, even if the roads were blocked, she could still make her way to the hospital. The main roads had been cleared the following morning and the journey to the hospital was uneventful, but the internal roads were impenetrable, blocked by three-foot-high drifts. The amazing thing about that conference was that forty-eight delegates arrived in Oswestry from schools as far flung as Dublin, Glasgow, Aberdeen, Bristol and London.[25] Oswestry was always a popular venue as accommodation was available on site and the conference catering was renowned. It was interesting to mingle with representatives from other schools and students particularly enjoyed the weekends.

The popularity of orthopaedic nursing as a precursor to the physiotherapy course had been reducing steadily since the 1967 intake and, although the school had been founded on the concept of combining the two courses for Oswestry-based students, it was time to reappraise the situation. Raising the academic pre-entry requirement to include a subject taken at Advanced level or, for Scottish applicants, two subjects taken at Higher level, was the final disincentive for candidates considering the dual qualification. Candidates were now expected to be at least eighteen years of age on leaving school and as such were eligible for direct entry to the physiotherapy course.

As the last students with any prior nursing experience had entered the school in 1974, it was decided in 1977, with some regrets, to discontinue combined training and in future to accept direct entrants only.

Two events of national importance to physiotherapy occurred during 1977, but their relevance and significance to the profession was not immediately recognised. The first was the publication of a Health Circular, HC77:33, which gave chartered physiotherapists the right to diagnose and treat disorders of function without prior referral by a doctor, dentist or veterinary surgeon. The circular initiated autonomous practice and gave physiotherapists the right to be first-contact practitioners. They were now empowered to generate their own workloads and were professionally responsible for their practice in designated areas, which gave them a higher level of autonomy than other paramedical practitioners in the UK and also a higher level of independence than other physical therapy professions throughout the world. The profession was relatively slow to embrace the full range of responsibilities presented by the Health Circular and it took some time for practitioners to develop the confidence to exploit the potential of their increased independence. By then, the professional body had developed an extensive network of practical, legal, moral and ethical guidelines to support independent practice.[26]

The second event, the introduction of a new course by the Teacher Training Subcommittee of the Education Committee of the CSP, had more direct application to the school. Marian Tidswell was respectively chair and member of the two CSP committees responsible for the development of the programme.[27] The course for the award of the Certificate in Education (Further Education) was the first educationally validated programme that accepted applications from chartered physiotherapists who held no other qualification. Teacher training now involved one year of study at a nominated college of further education to gain the Certificate, followed by a period of supervised teaching practice in a school for professional orientation prior to assessment and grading as a qualified teacher.

Accommodation and facilities of the school had been, for many years, totally inadequate to support the range of topics studied and the numbers of students passing through the course. Although locker accommodation was provided in Stoke-on-Trent at the Limes where the classrooms were located, there was no provision of similar facilities in the hospitals where clinical education was undertaken and students had no secure place to keep their personal belongings while they were working with patients. The theft of a student's purse while she was occupied with a patient on one of the wards brought matters to a head. CSP recommendations for student accommodation and other school requirements were again circulated to members of the Education Committee. Although members reluctantly agreed that the school's facilities fell short of the recommendations at both school bases, they identified there was little likelihood of major change in the foreseeable future. NSAHA representatives covered their perceived indifference to the school's problems by commenting

159

that the recommendations referred to an 'ideal' situation and, as there was an acute shortage of space at the NSRI, it was unlikely that any accommodation improvements could be provided.[28]

The problems were reinforced by the loss of the students' changing room facilities at the Limes in 1980, when they were commandeered for use as additional office accommodation. Hospital management suggested that this was to be a temporary situation, but it was feared that the loss would be permanent.[29] A feasibility study undertaken to determine action that could be taken to ease the accommodation problems was reported to the April 1980 Education Committee.[30] The study identified that the cost of essential improvement to the school was in the region of £10,000. As no capital development monies were available that year, the project would be carried forward for consideration as a priority for the following year.[31]

Accommodation continued to cause concern at Stoke-on-Trent as, one day in 1977, the classrooms at the Limes were locked and the keys removed. In consequence, teaching space was reduced to the entrance hall and stairs of the building, which posed health and safety hazards and inconvenience to the office workers based there. The situation remained unexplained and unresolved for several weeks, but eventually it transpired that social workers who had required additional storage space for home loan equipment had moved in without authorisation or communication with the school or hospital administration.[32] By April 1978, the teaching accommodation had been restored, but students had lost their changing facilities to nursing staff.[33]

Following repeated requests and letters of support from the CSP to the school's Education Committee, the AMT in Shropshire finally agreed that the school should have full-time secretarial support. Funding secretarial services was rated by the school as having a higher priority than supporting the student teacher's post[34] and Mrs Janet Lymn was appointed full-time secretary to the school with the money to pay her additional salary raised by withdrawal of financial support of the student teacher position. The negative aspect of this arrangement was that any subsequent recruitment of student teachers to the school would depend on the ability of the AHA to fund the post.[35] It was obvious that the post would never attract the priority level required for funding, as it would now be in direct competition with other projects that were readily identifiable as being of more immediate benefit to patients.

By 1978, the new curriculum was fully implemented and students attending the 'old' course had completed training or left the hospital. As the new course was organised within 'academic' years, students would not be in the hospitals during August. Oswestry was accustomed to a student presence throughout the year and requested that Wyn altered the 'new' course to maintain continuous clinical cover, but she refused. Staff referred to the 'contribution made by students to the clinical workload of the department', but the financial implications of the replacement of students by qualified staff appeared to be of more concern than the provision of an acceptable learning environment for the students.[36] Wyn was in sympathy with staff holiday cover problems but argued that, if the school was to continue to produce physiotherapists of a high standard and maintain the reputation of the hospital, it was imperative to give top priority to the students' educational needs.[37] The new course presented necessary educational progression for physiotherapists as, for the first time ever, they were identified as being supernumerary to the workforce rather than, as previously, being identified as trainees.

Following publication of the Sex Discrimination Act 1975, schools accepting female students only were obliged to review their recruitment policies. Oswestry had theoretically accepted male candidates for the combined orthopaedic nurse training/physiotherapy course between 1948 and 1954 while affiliated with the Royal Hospital Wolverhampton, but during those six years only one male candidate had been accepted and subsequently, by default, the school had reverted to a female-only intake. Section 29 of the Act identified physiotherapy schools as being in the position of persons 'concerned with the provision of goods, facilities or services to the public'. As such, it would be unlawful and contrary to the provisions of the Act for them to discriminate in the selection of students on the grounds of sex, unless such discrimination could be justified under the terms of the exceptions set out in Sections 35 and 46.

The Oswestry accommodation was totally inadequate for the numbers of students and staff using the school as there were no toilet, changing or washing facilities and students changed uniforms for practical or theoretical sessions in a curtained-off portion of a corridor outside one of their classrooms. As student changing facilities at both Stoke-on-Trent and Oswestry were virtually non-existent, Wyn used Section 35 of the Act as her reason for not recruiting male candidates. This section 'permits facilities and services to be restricted to one sex in certain situations where it is reasonable to do so in order to preserve decency and privacy'. She also stated that if the required facilities were made available to the school, she would be happy to recruit male candidates.[38]

No further action was contemplated as any change to existing arrangements would highlight the poverty of student provision at both branches of the school and the AHAs did not welcome any such exposure. The DHSS, however, responded by stating that the reasons the ONSSP had submitted to explain their restrictive recruitment policy would not be accepted as an adequate defence under the Act, 'at least over an extended period of time'. It was identified that, as many schools had embraced the new legislation, Oswestry was now one of the last eight to recruit female students only.[39] A scheme to convert the existing female physiotherapy toilet block in the main corridor to a male toilet and changing area was proposed, which would prove the school was accessible for students of both sexes, on paper at least.[40] However, the scheme did not progress and was never implemented.

In the meantime, the limited and sometimes inappropriate equipment at Stoke-on-Trent was causing Tony Fowler considerable frustration as he settled into his new post. He persuaded hospital administrators to acknowledge that it was dangerous practice to use metal plinths for the students' practise of electrotherapy techniques. Burns or electric shocks could result from models resting on a conducting surface when they were receiving short wave diathermy treatments or were using other electrical apparatus. This was a serious health hazard and wooden plinths were bought immediately to replace the metal ones.[41]

Owing to the financial stringency affecting Salop AHA, it was proposed that the Authority would no longer fund student or staff attendance at courses outside the region. This move was rejected by the Education Committee which was concerned that the specialised and isolated nature of the hospital and school in relation to the other physiotherapy schools required special consideration.[42] The question was mainly academic; however, as most courses attended by teaching staff had been self-financed for several years. It was reported to the same meeting that one of the teachers had completed a self-funded BA with the Open University and was now undertaking a (funded) middle management day release course at Cauldon College, Stoke-on-Trent.[43]

Physiotherapy schools are submitted to regular inspection to ensure that the required standards are being maintained. Initially these reviews were carried out by the CSP alone, but, after formation of the statutory body in 1960, they became the CPSM's responsibility with the CSP in attendance. The CPSM had failed to maintain the established quinquennial cycle of inspection with the result that several schools had not been visited for about seven or eight years. Wyn notified the Education Committee that she was to retire from post in August 1980 and reminded them that, as the last CPSM/CSP inspection had been conducted in 1974, prior to her appointment as principal, the school should be inspected before she retired.[44]

Following this inspection on 5–6 May 1981, the Education Committee received an advance copy of the report of the visit and was shocked to discover that the Physiotherapists' Board was seriously concerned about the future viability of the school. The committee was justly critical of the CPSM for not having arranged the visit earlier in Wyn's incumbency and felt strongly that, as visits were so far behind schedule, it would have been better to have delayed the inspection until after her retirement. They were devastated by the detail of the report which they felt had not been tempered with any sense of justice and considered that many of the comments made were harsh, unfair and unjust, particularly as the school's examination results tended to be higher than the national average. They considered that the inspectors had taken no account of the financial climate in the NHS since 1974. As the other four regionally based schools were modern and well equipped with excellent facilities for both students and staff, this comment was not based on the evidence.[45] Anne Steele, the newly appointed superintendent physiotherapist at North Staffordshire Royal Infirmary, welcomed the comments about staffing levels. She waged a constant battle for additional staff with hospital administration, but her carefully documented requests were always refused. The statutory body had now also identified the problem and this added weight to her future petitions and, eventually, she was able to appoint additional staff to the departments in Stoke-on-Trent.

The school was in the throes of a very severe staffing crisis as Jean Rogers and Bobbie Goff were rapidly approaching retirement age; Ralph Kay had contracted to work only one day a week; Pat Wood was to leave at the end of September; Tony Fowler had already left. There were in fact more vacancies on the teaching establishment than staff in post and the school was in an incredibly vulnerable position. The losses were marginally offset by Jean Davies, who had applied to undertake two terms' supervised teaching practice prior to the award of the Diploma of Teacher of Physiotherapy.[46]

Wyn had successfully introduced the new CSP Diploma course, and had coped with the problems of running a split-site school under difficult circumstances and the consequences of implementation of the Halsbury Report recommendations. Sadly, her many achievements were virtually eliminated by the devastating CPSM inspection report at the end of her time as principal. Despite the difficulties she experienced in the working environment, she retained a generosity of spirit and sense of humour that was latterly only obvious during her few off-duty hours.

NOTES

[1] Lord Halsbury, *Report of the Committee of Inquiry into the Pay and Related Conditions of Service of the Professions Supplementary to Medicine*, 1975

[2] Walton, J., ed., *The Oxford Companion to Medicine Vol. 2 N–Z*, Oxford, Oxford University Press, 1986

[3] '*Administration and Financing of Schools of Physiotherapy*', CPSM, 29 March 1973

[4] Extracts from the minutes of the ONSSP Education Committee meeting, 12 July 1973

[5] Extracts from the minutes of the ONSSP Education Committee meeting, 24 July 1978

[6] Extracts from the minutes of the ONSSP Education Committee meeting, 4 December 1978

[7] Berridge, J., *A Suitable Case for Treatment: A Case Study*, Milton Keynes, The Open University Press, 1976

[8] Lord Halsbury, *Report of the Committee of Inquiry into the Pay and Related Conditions of Service of the Professions Supplementary to Medicine*, 1975

[9] Houghton, *Report of the Committee of Inquiry into the Pay of Non-University Teachers*, December 1974

[10] *Shortage of Physiotherapy Teachers*, CSP Education Committee, October 1975

[11] Extracts from the minutes of the ONSSP Education Committee meeting, 26 September 1977

[12] Extracts from the minutes of the ONSSP Education Committee meeting, 20 July 1978

[13] Clegg, *Report of the Standing Committee on Pay and Comparability of Paramedical Professions*, 1979

[14] Extracts from the minutes of the ONSSP Education Committee meeting, 14 April 1980

[15] Extracts from the minutes of the ONSSP Education Committee meeting, 22 September 1975

[16] Extracts from the minutes of the ONSSP Education Committee meeting, 10 February 1975

[17] Extracts from the report of the CPSM Inspection, 5–6 May 1981

[18] Extracts from the minutes of the ONSSP Education Committee meeting, 12 May 1975

[19] Ibid

[20] Extracts from the minutes of the ONSSP Education Committee meeting, 27 September 1977

[21] Extracts from the minutes of the ONSSP Education Committee meeting, 12 January 1981

[22] Extracts from the minutes of the ONSSP Education Committee meeting, 24 July 1979

[23] Extracts from the minutes of the ONSSP Education Committee meeting, 22 September 1975

[24] Extracts from the report of the CPSM Inspection, 5–6 May 1981

[25] Extracts from the minutes of the ONSSP Education Committee meeting, 9 April 1979

[26] Tidswell, M., 'Physiotherapy: A True Profession?', unpublished MA dissertation, 1991

[27] Certificate in Education and Diploma of Teaching of Physiotherapy (Cert. in Ed. Dip TP)

[28] Extracts from the minutes of the ONSSP Education Committee meeting, 27 September 1977

[29] Extracts from the minutes of the ONSSP Education Committee meeting, 10 December 1979

[30] Extracts from the minutes of the ONSSP Education Committee meeting, 14 April 1980

[31] Extracts from the minutes of the ONSSP Education Committee meeting, 12 January 1981

[32] Extracts from the minutes of the ONSSP Education Committee meeting, 27 September 1977

[33] Extracts from the minutes of the ONSSP Education Committee meeting, 10 April 1978

[34] Extracts from the minutes of the ONSSP Education Committee meeting, 12 December 1977

[35] Extracts from the minutes of the ONSSP Education Committee meeting, 27 September 1977

[36] Extracts from the minutes of the ONSSP Education Committee meeting, 11 December 1978

[37] Extracts from the minutes of the ONSSP Education Committee meeting, 4 December 1978

[38] Extracts from the minutes of the ONSSP Education Committee meeting, 9 April 1979

[39] Extracts from the minutes of the ONSSP Education Committee meeting, 24 July 1979

[40] Extracts from the minutes of the ONSSP Education Committee meeting, 4 December 1978

[41] Extracts from the minutes of the ONSSP Education Committee meeting, 9 April 1979

[42] Extracts from the minutes of the ONSSP Education Committee meeting, 24 July 1979

[43] Extracts from the minutes of the ONSSP Education Committee meeting, 12 January 1981

[44] Ibid

[45] Extracts from the minutes of the ONSSP Education Committee meeting, 29 June 1981

[46] Extracts from the minutes of the ONSSP Education Committee meeting, 17 August 1981

Chapter 12
A Time of Renewal: 1981–1983

Years of underinvestment in the infrastructure of the school by both funding Health Authorities, combined with lack of internal drive to recruit teachers to replace the experienced staff approaching retirement, had, by the CPSM inspection in May 1981, brought the school to its nadir. Compounded by the failure to respond effectively to recommendations in earlier inspection reports, the level of personnel and financial resources now required to enable the school to meet all CPSM/CSP standards by 1986 was realistically beyond the capability of the two funding Health Authorities to satisfy. The sensible decision would have been to close the school following the 1981 CPSM inspection and to relocate existing students to alternative institutions to complete their studies.

The report had identified that, despite its physical deficits, the programme implemented by the school maintained the development of a high degree of clinical competence and confidence in course participants who were received enthusiastically by hospitals throughout the country on qualification. This may have been the deciding factor that persuaded the Health Authorities to support it for another two years when they interviewed for the principal's post in July.

When shown the CPSM report on the morning of the interviews, Marian Tidswell had not sufficient time to digest the contents fully, but on this first reading felt the comments in regard to accommodation and facilities were fair and accurate. Holding this view she found herself at variance with the opinions of the interview panel, however; when invited to comment she used the example of the accommodation at Stoke-on-Trent to respond to the specific question. In the room dedicated to theory teaching at the Limes, fifteen students were taught with fourteen desks and thirteen chairs and the practical classroom was so small that the student group could not all cram into the room in standing, let alone sit down and use apparatus. Accommodation was a very obvious defect of the school and the panel did not address any other areas commented on in the report.

Marian was appointed to the post and spent the next seven weeks planning and preparing her initial approaches to the challenges ahead. She was assured of total support from staff and students, and immediately introduced a framework for dialogue that would keep everyone concerned fully informed of the school's situation. It was believed that this enhanced communication between staff and students would help invalidate the rumours rampant in the hospital, defuse the tension that existed and give everyone the opportunity to receive correct, up-to-date information regarding the school's current position. This open-door policy was a valuable innovation and was to reap many benefits at a later date when the need for mutual trust and confidence was much needed.

She developed a five-year plan with specific goals to be achieved by six, twenty-two and fifty-eight months; the expected times of her initial review and possible confirmation in post, the CPSM interim inspection and the next full CPSM inspection. Although daunted by the magnitude of the task ahead, she was quite well prepared and, although lacking in managerial experience, had a theoretical understanding of the CPSM's requirements. She was cautiously optimistic of a final positive result as full cooperation was promised and subsequently freely given by the two Health Authorities, who were understandably less optimistic. The main priority initially was to maintain course teaching for existing students and for those about to enter the course, with possibly only three staff in post. This was closely followed by the need to address in turn the recommendations of the May CPSM inspection report.

Three specific recommendations had been identified in the report. The first permitted the school to continue until an interim inspection two years ahead would review the changes implemented by the new principal and assess if sufficient progress had been made to allow its continuance to the next scheduled quinquennial visit. The second and third recommendations were linked. The numbers of students accepted annually for the course was to be reduced to twenty from the 1982 intake and any last-minute cancellations for 1981 were not to be replaced. This reduced the 1981 cohort to twenty-seven from the initial thirty accepted for the course.[1]

In addition, six areas were highlighted as requiring urgent attention. They had been addressed comprehensively in the body of the report and provided a framework about which activities were necessarily to be planned. They were:

1. Recognition of the geographical and educational isolation of the school coupled with the need for radical realignment of the school's educational philosophy.
2. The need for urgent exploration of all possible links with higher education with active pursuit of the best option.
3. Reappraisal of the course plan and its redesign to ensure correlation of theoretical and clinical components.
4. Reassessment of the clinical staffing levels at Oswestry and Stoke-on-Trent to ensure that students were supernumerary to the workforce.
5. Changes in organisation to achieve greater participation by students, teachers and clinicians in the running of the school.
6. Adequate financial provision to ensure that the proposals identified throughout the report could be implemented.[2]

A simple course plan was devised for students arriving in September 1981 and the syllabi for the second- and third-year students reviewed and rearranged to ensure required course components would be completed within specified time schedules. At this stage, it was not possible to eliminate the duplication of classroom teaching involved in operating the split site; however, simple reordering of the clinical education enabled students to maximise their benefit of the wealth of clinical experience available. Owing to the staffing situation, teachers were obliged to accept classroom contact with students far in excess of the recommended twenty hours a week and it was only with their abundant goodwill and long experience that implementation of the proposed course teaching schedules was possible.

It was recognised that, in an ideal situation, students' educational expectations would be realised and teachers' academic aspirations satisfied, but the funding arrangements for NHS-based professional education had created a less than ideal situation. Both funding Health Authorities of the school had major though different financial problems. Shropshire had no medical school or university within the county boundaries to encourage investment in education and had a low-density population scattered in villages and small market towns over a wide geographical area, with a disproportionately large population in the southern end of the county in new town development. North Staffordshire supported the largest population of all the West Midland Region's Health Authorities. A century or more of work in the coal mines and pottery industry in Stoke-on-Trent had produced a population with a substantially higher than normal incidence of chronic respiratory problems. In both Health Authorities, the per capita cost of basic health care provision was higher than in many other areas of the country and financial hardship was evident in these areas before it was obvious elsewhere in the NHS. For the Authorities to commit to the support of the school under these circumstances was surprising as the resources required would stretch their already tight budgets to the limit.

When appraised of the detail of the SAHA school budget, retention of the hitherto underused budget lines was immediately negotiated as the approach to budget management was clearly defined – the specified department could either use allocated resources by the end of each financial year or lose them. Any budget allocations unspent by early April were returned to the common financial pool and eliminated from subsequent budget statements. Overspends were dealt with in a similar manner. If a department exceeded its budget allocations in any one area, the amount of overspend was deducted from subsequent allocations.

Requests for priority funds were submitted to the Salop Area Management Team which amounted to £30,000 for upgrading the accommodation, £12,500 for the replacement of electrical equipment, £5,000 for the supply of books and teaching aids, and finally some £2,000 for upgrading of some furnishings within the school.[3] These monies, if awarded, were to be allocated, at the latest, within the 1982/1983 financial year.

The most glaring defects of the school identified by the 1981 CPSM inspection were the lack of appropriate teaching equipment, teaching aids and accommodation for both students and staff. In Shropshire, the identified budget allocation was £546 for teaching equipment and £158 for textbooks and publications. Additionally textbooks could be ordered through the librarian at Oswestry and the supplies officer at Stoke-on-Trent.[4] Inspectors had expressed their concern that even this limited allocation had not been spent, in view of the obvious and urgent need at both school bases.

The CPSM had identified that 'the existing level of provision was inadequate for the number of students in the school and much of the equipment for student use was outdated'.[5] In fact the only short wave diathermy machine that would tune effectively was obsolete. It was valve operated and as such was so outdated it was excluded from the annual equipment service agreements. This machine, when new, had been saved from the 1948 fire that destroyed the school buildings and most of the equipment, but now its days were numbered for safety reasons.

Another teaching aid rescued from the fire was a papier maché model of a torso with detachable organs. By 1981, after generations of fumbling student use, the organs would fit in any chosen position and it was also of little further practical use in the classroom. A skeleton donated in the early '70s by a grateful parent and an ancient slide projector received from the school of nursing on their purchase of a more recent model completed the list of teaching aids available for use in the school.

The inspectors recommended the provision of duplicating/photocopying equipment, access to appropriate visual aids for teaching, purchase of modern short wave diathermy and muscle stimulating apparatus, and provision of library shelving and multiple copies of essential texts.[6] These items were the responsibility of the Health Authority to provide. Jeff Silk, Secretary to the

Education Committee and Sector Administrator of the Northern Sector of Salop Health Authority, guided Marian through all negotiations and cleared the path to the appropriate members of the two Health Authorities.

Salop Area Management Team confirmed their allocation of £12,500 for improvement to the school's electrical and movement equipment and also awarded £4,000 for minor alterations to provide seminar rooms.[7] The first lists of essential equipment required were produced and justified with Jeff Silk's assistance and orders placed before Christmas 1981. By the end of the financial year, £500 of this money was lost, as not all ordered items were received by the deadline. The school's benefit was reduced to the £12,000 spent on the electrical and other equipment supplied and delivered in time. This was a very generous amount to be awarded to a department that was not concerned directly with patient care; however, in the event of the school's closure in 1983, the new equipment could be redistributed to needy physiotherapy departments across the Health Authority.

Negotiations were also initiated with the League of Friends of the Hospital to secure the significant improvements required in the school's teaching equipment that fell outwith and were in excess of the Health Authority's financial allocations. The League recognised that if the school was to continue to compete in the field of professional education, it required additional equipment to facilitate student learning and encourage in-depth study and research. As the Health Authority could not consider such items as valid use of their limited resources, they came to the school's rescue.[8]

Between 1981 and 1984 the various branches of the League of Friends of the Robert Jones and Agnes Hunt Orthopaedic Hospital donated a staggering £15,207 to the Oswestry school base. It was used to purchase overhead projectors, a range of anatomical models, textbooks, tape/slide projectors and video equipment. This unprecedented level of support helped secure the school's future at the 1983 inspection, enabling the demonstration of the provision of the normal range of teaching equipment expected in a school of physiotherapy. Students also contributed to further purchases when they donated the £400 raised by a sponsored disco to buy traction equipment.

The 1981 report stated that teaching accommodation at Oswestry was inadequate and somewhat fragmented; at Stoke-on-Trent, it was described as being entirely inadequate.[9] Urgent action was required, particularly at Stoke-on-Trent where, for more than a decade, staff and students had battled with unsatisfactory and steadily deteriorating facilities. It was predicted that the accommodation problems would continue to be insurmountable and so it was a pleasant surprise when a more suitable venue for the North Staffordshire component of the school was identified at the Nurses' Home of the Haywood Hospital at Tunstall, Stoke-on-Trent. The facility was now surplus to the Authority's requirements and had become available at the most opportune time. Little alteration was required to make a useful classroom, study, common room, residential accommodation for students and an office for teaching staff. It would however be more than a year from the move when the £1,000 allocated by North Staffordshire Area Health Authority to complete the alterations was made available and put to use.[10] When the chalk boards, suspension frames, wall bars and notice boards were finally fixed to walls and ceilings, the school base was very impressive.

Prior to the move it was decided that, as students were to be resident in the same building as their teaching accommodation, they would be able to use these areas for evening study. They were supplied with keys to the library and the classroom and were responsible for the security of the building's study facilities. Apart from occasional lost keys, the system worked well and few losses of books or equipment were reported.

One bright frosty day during February 1982, Jean Davies, Janet Lymn and Marian Tidswell closed the school at the Limes, packed everything into boxes and supervised the loading of removal vans.[11] The vans led the way to Tunstall, followed by the three members of staff who then unpacked the new facility. Although the Health Authority had paid for the hire of the removal vans, they were unable to provide manpower for the packing and unpacking of the equipment.

On the first of several trips to the Haywood Hospital from the

Limes, Janet and Marian followed one of the vans, but the second time they attempted the journey without this guidance they became hopelessly lost, covering many unnecessary miles before any landmark was recognised. It was Janet's first visit to the school base and she recognised during her brief time there the reasons for many of the complaints she had heard from teaching staff over the years. The new school base was approximately seven miles from the hospitals in which students gained clinical experience, but this was a relatively minor problem readily solved by the provision of hospital transport.[12]

The accommodation improvements required at Oswestry were a culmination of the issues raised repeatedly in previous inspection reports that had been collectively reiterated in 1981. Once again it had been stated that students and staff required adequate study/library areas, an additional class/seminar room, storage space, preparation areas adjacent to practical rooms and changing facilities for students within the school to include toilet and shower facilities.[13] During the early months of the principal's incumbency, there were many discussions with the Salop Area Management Team followed by the preparation of plans for accommodation improvements at Oswestry and, on this occasion, action followed some months behind that taken by North Staffordshire Area Health Authority.

Throughout 1982 and well into the following year, the £30,000 awarded by Salop Area Management Team was put to good use and the Oswestry base of the school was dusty, cluttered and physically disorganised as workmen moved systematically through the building, upgrading and refurbishing. Although an attempt was made to complete the work over the school's summer break, this was not possible and, once teaching recommenced in September, workmen, staff and students were all competing for the same space as they tried to complete their allotted tasks. There was no quiet corner of the school and staff voices rose steadily over time to overcome the pneumatic drills that accompanied each class.

When not teaching, staff wandered around distractedly, each clutching a cardboard box in which was stored teaching notes, papers to mark, agendas and minutes of meetings, and anything else considered necessary to ensure survival over the many months of disruption. Their working lives had been reduced to the contents of this one portable cardboard box and this provided the lifeline for each teacher throughout the months of school alterations.

Every part of the school was subjected to upgrading or change of use and, on completion of the work, the original student reference library had become a second teachers' room and the secretary's office and that of the principal had had structural alterations to make them more work-friendly. These three rooms were also carpeted and decorated. The original teachers' room was carpeted and curtained but redecoration was abandoned after a wait of several months. The furniture was repositioned and staff returned to their little-changed room in order to regain some semblance of normality.

The staff changing room was transformed into the students' library and was immediately put to full use, much to the relief of the hospital medical staff who were able once more to secure a place in the medical library. The staff changing facilities displaced by the upgrading were moved to the area previously used by occupational therapy staff of the hospital and the changing facilities for all female students were relocated to their previously identified common room.

Male students, who had been sharing little more than a cupboard with occupational therapy technical instructors, were now accommodated in the cloakroom previously occupied by second-year students located behind the League of Friends Hospital Shop. The original cloakroom for third-year students, also at a distance from the main hospital building, was returned to the general accommodation pool of the hospital. The final change was the provision of two seminar rooms and a common room in an area that had been a gardener's cottage. This final accommodation provision gave students further areas for private study and also provided facilities for small group teaching. Further proposals included the conversion of the former assistant principal's office to an audio-visual library/study, which was completed during 1983.

All was completed by July 1983 and at the CPSM interim

inspection the inspectors commented that they were impressed with the progress made by the school, particularly as it had been achieved not only at a time of financial stringency but also against the background of further NHS reorganisation.[14] Particular mention was made of the refurbishment of the offices, creation of a school library and audio-visual study room, provision of a students' common room, changing accommodation and cloakrooms.[15]

Another of the issues raised by the 1981 CPSM inspection report had been the educational isolation of the school and it had recommended that links with higher education establishments be strengthened.[16] The case presented by the CSP to the Minister of State for Social Security in 1981 suggesting that physiotherapy should be a graduate entry profession had met with a negative response. The Minister had indicated that the government would not fund this development and courses developed would have to be funded by the Health Authorities in which the schools were based.[17] The most promising venue for a degree course was Chester College, a degree awarding body of Liverpool University. During the first year in post, Marian negotiated and planned a course that was appropriate for professional needs, could be conducted between Chester College and Oswestry, and would cost approximately £1,500 per student per course to implement.

Chester recognised physiotherapy as an educationally deprived profession with students and staff of the school demonstrating an academic profile that was well above university minimal entry requirements. The college offered school staff equivalent status in the university to that awarded in the NHS. Unfortunately, Chester lies outside the West Midlands region and, although nearer to Oswestry than the Stoke-on-Trent base of the school, the additional costs for implementation of the course could not be considered.[18]

Stoke-on-Trent expressed a preference for consideration of a similar project development with the North Staffordshire Polytechnic or Keele University. These proposals did not progress as neither institution could offer the facilities required by the course in specific subject areas of expertise, nor could they supply the required accommodation needs.[19] Discussions were discontinued in June 1982.

Restructuring of the clinical education programme was essential and was addressed within the first few months of the principal's appointment. The situation was simplified initially by eliminating the split day at Oswestry. By arranging for students to gain experience in complete half days, rather than having occasional classes interspersed with patient contact, they were immediately more motivated, the scheduling of academic components was eased and there was more flexibility in the system. At Stoke-on-Trent, student clinical hours were extended to give longer exposure to the medical and surgical experience not available at Oswestry. This had the effect of reducing the amount of time in school, but was considered by students to be of benefit to their overall education.

Clinical staff, particularly at Stoke-on-Trent, worked with enthusiasm to assist the school to produce placement-specific objectives of clinical practice, circulated prior to the start of each secondment so that both student and staff expectations were known in advance of attendance. Subsequently, in preparation of the clinical rotas, it was ensured students gained a progressive clinical education appropriate for a pre-registration course, with placement requirements tailored to their individual needs.

This was the most satisfying part of the necessary work at this time as it confirmed the range and quality of experience available for student learning. Stoke-on-Trent offered students the opportunity to treat patients with a range of medical chest conditions that was unrivalled by any other area of the country and the quality of the orthopaedic experience at Oswestry was legendary. Informing staff appropriately of the level of previous knowledge and skills gained by students prior to their attendance on the placement was a constructive move that eliminated much of the previous tension. Students and staff now knew precisely what was expected of them, both were prepared adequately for placements and the previous uncertainties apparent in the unfamiliar settings were largely eliminated.

Students provided clinical cover for fifty-one weeks of the year and during the second and third years of the course worked alternate Saturday mornings. Initial attempts to change these systems highlighted the extremely low establishments of qualified physiotherapy staff in both Health Authorities and confirmed the extent of the student contribution to the maintenance of the standard of patient care provided. It was also recognised that students had educational needs in the clinical environment and staffing levels did not allow clinical teaching to be carried out effectively.

After long discussion and hard negotiation at Oswestry a compromise solution was reached. Saturday mornings were readily surrendered, but the reduction of student cover during the vacations was fiercely contested. August cover had already been reduced slightly by the introduction of the revised course. Since 1978, the only students available were those who had failed one or more components of the Part 2 qualifying examination as they returned to Oswestry to complete their studies during the second half of the month. Eventually, reluctant agreement was achieved and all student contact with clinical areas was eliminated for eight weeks of the year, allowing complete sets of students to take annual leave, rather than the set being split to provide continuous clinical cover. With the previous arrangements, teaching staff had experienced difficulty in arranging annual leave owing to teaching and clinical supervision commitments, but, as reduction of the clinical cover by seven weeks also reduced teaching contact by the same amount, they now also had improved choice. More radical plans for restructuring the course programme were delayed until the outcome of the 1983 CPSM inspection was known.

The extreme vulnerability of the school was evident in the staffing position as by the end of September, the staff/student ratio had risen to 1:26, significantly at variance with the CSP recommendation of 1:12. This situation caused continuing concern and would take several years to resolve. With significant recruitment, however, and the supportive effect of the mandatory reduction in student intake, the staff/student ratios were steadily reduced and by January 1985 finally achieved the higher education recommendation of 1:10.

At the start of the 1981–2 academic year, only Marian, Jean Rogers, Bobbie Goff and Jean Davies, a new student teacher, were in full-time posts, Ralph Kay was working one day only each week and Pat Wood had already left to take up a post at the

Withington School of Physiotherapy. Margaret Green and Mr Simpson taught the gym sessions at Oswestry and Stoke-on-Trent respectively and, for a few months, Nora Richards, a qualified teacher and former student of the school, worked a few hours each week. The course could maintain its dubious viability solely by being supported by the CSP national examination system. Jean, Bobbie and Marian shared the majority of the teaching, Ralph retained responsibility for electrotherapy until his final departure from the NHS in April 1982 and Jean Davies started her new career by teaching parts of the movement syllabus, mentored by Bobbie and Jean.

The school had previously lost funding for its student teacher post, unoccupied for seven years, by the authorised virement of the budget line to fund, in part, the salary of the full-time school secretary. There was now a danger of losing funding for some of the unoccupied establishment teaching posts; however, the Health Authorities willingly agreed to retain them all so that recruitment of appropriate teaching staff would not be inhibited. They also agreed to retain the school's training budget, which was to prove very helpful in encouraging the recruitment and retention of potential teachers of the calibre required to carry the school forward. This enabled the appointment of more student teachers than were permitted by the establishment, funding them from the unoccupied qualified teacher posts, and was of immediate encouragement to existing school personnel. The flexibility these measures allowed was a significant boost to recruitment of the precious teaching resource.

The physiotherapy profession was, in the early 1980s, slowly coming to terms with the extent of the responsibility and freedom that resulted from first-contact practice initiated by implementation of the Health Circular HC77:33 and few courses, as yet, addressed the extended professional role effectively. First-contact practice and improved levels of professional competence in the clinical field demanded additional individual specialist input to the curriculum to prepare course qualifiers adequately for the enhanced professional roles and responsibilities of the modern clinical practitioner.

Marian, Bobbie and Jean were experienced teachers with clinical specialism in orthopaedics, trauma and rheumatology. Bobbie offered, in addition, exceptional clinical knowledge, experience and expertise in neurology. During the 1960s, before undertaking her physiotherapy training, Jean Davies, a qualified teacher of gymnastics, had taught educational and remedial gymnastics to the students and was therefore, with her dual qualification and experience, able to make an immediate significant contribution to course teaching[20] and volunteered to take an interest in movement studies. With this basic team, supported by Ralph and Nora, the school could survive for a few months if ultimate improvement in the situation was visualised.

Years of experience at Oswestry and cognisance of the staffing position in all NHS-based schools determined from the outset that recruitment of student teachers was likely to be more successful than that of qualified staff. Under normal circumstances a principal was not allowed to train student teachers until two years after appointment, but as Marian had developed and implemented the CSP teacher-training course followed since 1977, she was not subjected to this restriction. She considered the most effective policy was to encourage recruitment of clinical experts from areas that would complement rather than supplement the existing expertise within the school.

Owing to staff shortages, she was not able to offer new student teachers the supportive environment they had a right to expect, but, with the training budget in place, she was able to offer funding support for postgraduate study. Few NHS-based schools were able to offer this opportunity to their staff at that time and it proved to be a factor that enabled recruitment of high-flying academic student teachers. They considered funding of postgraduate study at such an early stage of the profession's educational development significantly outweighed the drudgery of taking a teaching load that was far in excess of recommended contact levels.

The school urgently required staff who had experience and expertise in research and the cardiovascular and respiratory areas of physiotherapy practice. Jean Davies fitted the research profile admirably as she had, on qualification, worked for some time in orthopaedics before moving to a physiotherapy research post –

among the first to be created nationwide, at the orthotic research and locomotor assessment unit (ORLAU) in the hospital. Approximately two years later, she was appointed to a second research post, this time in the spinal disorders unit. These unique specialist units had been established at Oswestry during the 1970s and were led by orthopaedic surgeon directors who developed multidisciplinary research teams to include physiotherapists. One of the most notable achievements of the spinal disorders unit during Jean's occupancy of the post was the development of the Oswestry Low Back Pain Disability Questionnaire.[21] It is still used worldwide to assess individual ability, evaluate the effectiveness of treatment and develop strategies for future management of the patient's condition. At Oswestry, based on the information obtained by the questionnaires, another former student, Else Goss, developed a schedule for the management of persistent back pain under the guise of the Functional Restoration Programme.[22]

As Pat Wood had been fully trained in Maitland Mobilisations, a replacement was urgently needed or this essential subject would be lost from the school's curriculum. Pat had been responsible for the teaching, clinical supervision and assessment of all students in this specialist field. A potential replacement was found when Phyl Fletcher-Cook, a qualified teacher, approached the school. She had trained at the Bradford Hospitals School of Physiotherapy, but could not be offered a position there on qualification and came to Oswestry in January 1982.[23] She possessed all the qualities hoped for in a new teacher; she was keen, enthusiastic and meticulous in her preparation and delivery of the syllabus, and was a welcome addition to the small staff. She immediately started the prolonged training to be the school's new Maitland Mobilisations expert and, with Jean Davies qualifying in March 1982, the staffing situation looked promising.

In September 1982, three student teachers were recruited of whom two were funded by unoccupied establishment teaching posts and one by the reinstated student teacher's post. Cath Rose, formerly a secondary school teacher, had trained as a physiotherapist at the ONSSP in the late 1970s. She followed in Jean Davies' footsteps and started the two-term assessment programme. Jill Humphreys and Jean Webb enrolled on the Certificate in Further Education/Diploma of Teaching Physiotherapy programme at Dudley College/ONSSP.[24] Although Jill was the only one of the three to offer significant expertise in areas not already covered by the existing staff, recruitment of the other two was considered essential to maintain the gruelling teaching schedules.

Jean Rogers retired from full-time work in December 1982. Her calmness in every crisis and her unstinting support and encouragement were sadly missed. She returned, however, almost immediately for two days a week during February and March 1983 to support the school through a period of extreme staff shortages compounded by a severe outbreak of flu.[25] Unfortunately, her replacement, Ruby Jeffers, came to the school in April 1983 and left for personal reasons in late May, despite expressing the highest regard for the principal, staff and students.

Ruby's resignation, coupled with Bobbie Goff's planned retirement in July and Jean Davies' absence through illness from April 1983 until October, returned the school to a very vulnerable position and once again put it at significant risk. Cath Rose and Phyl Fletcher-Cook were proving to be valuable assets, but they lacked the necessary experience to take the teaching load that had been carried by Jean Rogers, Bobbie Goff and Marian Tidswell over the past two years. Staff were stretched to the absolute limit[26] and hoped the burden would be eased when the student teachers qualified in December.

Staff recruitment was buoyant although actual numbers of staff in post had only marginally improved by the time of the CPSM interim inspection in July 1983. The inspectors commented that there had been a significant improvement in the educational process in the school since the previous inspection and a nucleus of keen teaching staff were in post.[27] They recognised that these achievements had resulted from individual hard work, but commented that the school would not achieve its full potential until a group of senior teaching staff were in post at both sites, to enable the principal to adopt the role of planner and coordinator.[28] It was believed that senior staff would appear in time, so they did not enforce the closure announced two years earlier. They indicated that the student intake could be increased to twenty-four when staffing levels permitted with senior staff in post at both school sites. Fortunately, neither the inspectors nor the school could predict that Jean Webb would return to clinical work without completing the teacher training course, and, although Jill Humphreys would qualify in December 1983, she would decide to devote her time to home and family, and not join the staff. Jean Davies would ultimately succumb to her illness and the future staffing position was bleak.

Throughout the first turbulent months of Marian's appointment, second- and third-year students were incredible. Their school was in chaos, there were few staff and the facilities, which had always been poor, deteriorated further before any improvement was effected. The students had many grounds for complaint, but these were never articulated. They seemed to appreciate staff efforts in difficult circumstances and voiced no criticism. Traditionally they invited teaching staff at Christmas to share mince pies and sherry before leaving for the Christmas break. It was the occasion for students to give staff a small present and the one they presented to Marian was greatly appreciated as it was a candle that could be burned at both ends!

Students appeared relaxed and lighthearted, supportive, cooperative and interested in everything that was going on. However, significant change is disruptive and the more advanced their studies, the more disruption major change produces. Students entering the third year of the course in September 1981 missed Wyn Cannell and Pat Wood far more strongly than the students following a year behind in the course. In addition to the 'normal' problems generated by the new teaching arrangements, they were also unsettled by the frequent appearance of white-shirted men bearing clipboards and tape measures, intent on recording the dimensions of the school for use by the next occupants.

Although the finalist students had been loyal, tolerant, apparently resilient, bright, positive and cooperative throughout the year, the results of their qualifying examinations were disappointing. They were no reflection of the students' ability nor rewarded their hard work over a very difficult period. Only ten of the twenty-six entrants to the examination qualified at the first attempt. Two had already deferred entry until November on health grounds and the remaining sixteen failed one or more component of the examination. By the November retake examinations, results presented a more normal achievement; the two first entry candidates qualified, as did fourteen of the sixteen re-entry students, leaving only two to enter the fourth year prior to their third and final attempt to qualify.

The students decided they should make more of a celebration of their qualification than had previous groups and the first of new-style badge-giving ceremonies took place in July 1982 with Ida Bromley, the Chairman of the CSP Council, travelling to Oswestry to present the badges. The following year, Jean Rogers and, in 1984, Bobbie Goff were invited and accepted the honour. It was fitting that the students, to whom Jean and Bobbie had dedicated so much of their lives, should honour them in this way.

These students and those who qualified in 1983 demonstrated a remarkable level of professional behaviour during the 1981–2 winter. When blizzards in early January caused havoc to road and rail transport across the country, second-year and finalist students on their own initiative, during the worst of the weather, clambered through thigh-high snowdrifts the four miles to and from the hospital to treat patients. They had been concerned that qualified staff were likely to be snowed up and unable to travel to work and put the patients' needs before their own comfort and safety in true Oswestry tradition. Later, the students due to qualify in 1983 were significantly disrupted by the building alterations within the school that would not benefit their own studies, but they welcomed the work, recognising it would improve conditions for future student cohorts.

They held a twenty-four-hour sponsored disco in the physiotherapy gymnasium during their final year, raising over £400 for equipment for the school. It was extremely well organised and a very private affair; all appropriate permissions had been granted and, with the fire door of the physiotherapy department closed, no sound escaped to the main corridor. Students had arranged for police checks throughout the night to ensure no uninvited people were in the hospital grounds and Marian worked in her office until 7 a.m. to give them added support. The first of several predicted complaints about the disco were received shortly after 8 a.m. Students were held responsible for a reported stampede of cows in a field close to the hospital, caused by the undue noise that had been generated. The noise was also reported to have kept children on Wheatley Ward awake. Patients in other wards apparently had been disturbed by all the comings and goings of 'undesirable' elements at all hours of the night. However, nothing was pursued once the complainants were informed that the principal had been on site throughout the night to ensure everything was conducted in an appropriate manner and, to her certain knowledge, nobody had been disturbed or inconvenienced.

The twenty-seven students entering the course in September 1981 arrived when Marian was still knocking on the door of her office before entering, having not yet become comfortable in her new role. Their time at Oswestry was punctuated by changes in all aspects of school life affecting course organisation, accommodation and personnel. The cohort included three young men – Adrian Nottingham, Stuart Nottingham and Keith Jeavons – and was the first intake to recognise that male candidates were welcome to apply to Oswestry. Initially, their changing accommodation was little more than a cupboard shared with OT technicians, too small to accommodate them all at the same time. Later, as numbers increased, more appropriate facilities were negotiated.

The first group of students to be selected for the course after the 1981 CPSM inspection entered in September 1982. Jean and Marian interviewed and offered places to the twenty-strong cohort during the autumn 1981 term. Neither of the interviewers had gained significant previous experience in this area of activity and they spent many hours agonising over their choices. They were usually more anxious and nervous than the candidates they interviewed. When the final choice was made, Jean commented that not only were the group of suitable academic ability to undertake the course successfully, but they also had the makings of a potentially fine orchestra. The cohort was a little light on the woodwind section but the strength of the strings was quite gratifying. When they arrived, it was apparent that it was not an orchestra that had been selected – the school had in fact acquired twenty soloists. Many people in the hospital commented that this cohort was of a different type from all previous groups and wrung their hands in despair for the future of the school, doubts not shared by the school nor by the students concerned. They were lively young people who coped with major staff shortages, building alterations and many other disruptions throughout the course, while attempting to complete their studies within normal timescales.

During 1982 there was a further reorganisation of the National Health Service aimed at simplifying management structures below regional level and achieving a ten per cent reduction in management costs. The ninety Area Health Authorities were abolished and replaced by 192 District Health Authorities (DHAs) directly accountable to the unaffected Regional Health Authorities. Each DHA now had a Multidisciplinary Team (MDT) that included nursing but not paramedical professions. District and Regional Multidisciplinary Teams had no accountability to each other; neither were individual officers accountable between the tiers. The DHA was accountable to the RHA while District and Regional Chairmen were directly accountable to the Secretary of State. Decisions were taken by consensus and officers in the team continued to carry individual responsibility for specified professional functions.

Initially there was little observable change in the management arrangements in the two Health Authorities supporting the school following this reorganisation. Marian found with relief that many of the people with whom she had been dealing over the previous two years were unchanged, although they were now operating under a different job title. One minor positive move was that the School Education Committee requested representation from the student body. This, combined with the staff/student meetings that had been established two years earlier, was a further boost to enhanced communication in the school and students took their responsibilities as disseminators of information from both these meetings very seriously.

A feature of the reorganisation was the development of a

management structure within the districts to include 'units' that could have, as in Shropshire, a geographical or functional basis. The system was very flexible – a single hospital or a locality with its catchment population, a defined psychiatric service or a comprehensive maternity service could all justify Unit status. The Unit Management Teams (UMT) consisted of an administrator, a nursing officer and a medical representative.[29]

The Health Authorities had given more active support to the school over the previous two years than had been evident at any other time in its history and were rewarded by the positive outcome of the interim inspection in July 1983. All the physical and philosophical improvements that had been made were recognised, but concern was expressed that, in addition to planning and coordinating, Marian maintained a heavy teaching load with no senior teaching staff in post and was attempting to rebuild the course with higher educational links.[30] Clear, effective channels of communication between district and unit administration and the principal at Stoke-on-Trent were required, as was a defined budget for the school with the principal as budget holder.[31]

NOTES

[1] Extracts from the report of the CPSM Inspection, 5–6 May 1981

[2] Ibid

[3] Extracts from the minutes of the ONSSP Education Committee meeting, 30 November 1981

[4] Extracts from the report of the CPSM Inspection, 5–6 May 1981

[5] Ibid

[6] Ibid

[7] Extracts from the minutes of the ONSSP Education Committee meeting, 26 February 1982

[8] Ibid

[9] Extracts from the report of the CPSM Inspection, 5–6 May 1981

[10] Extracts from the minutes of the ONSSP Education Committee meeting, 26 February 1982

[11] Ibid

[12] Extracts from the minutes of the ONSSP Education Committee meeting, 28 September 1982

[13] Extracts from the report of the CPSM Inspection, 5–6 May 1981

[14] Extracts from the report of the CPSM Interim Inspection, 11–12 July 1983

[15] Ibid

[16] Extracts from the report of the CPSM Inspection, 5–6 May 1981

[17] Barclay, Jean, *In Good Hands,* Chapter 11, p.274, Oxford, Butterworth Heinemann Ltd, 1994

[18] Extracts from the minutes of the ONSSP Education Committee meeting, 23 March 1982

[19] Extracts from the minutes of the ONSSP Education Committee meeting, 2 July 1982

[20] Extracts from the minutes of the ONSSP Education Committee meeting, 28 September 1981

[21] Fairbank, J.C.T., Coupar, J., Davies, J.B. and O'Brien, J., 'The Oswestry Low Back Pain Disability Questionnaire', *Physiotherapy* Vol. 66 no. 8, p.271–273

[22] Tidswell, M.E., *Orthopaedic Physiotherapy*, London, Mosby International Ltd, 1998

[23] Extracts from the minutes of the ONSSP Education Committee meeting, 2 July 1982

[24] Extracts from the minutes of the ONSSP Education Committee meeting, 4 November 1982

[25] Extracts from the minutes of the ONSSP Education Committee meeting, 19 May 1983

[26] Extracts from the minutes of the ONSSP Education Committee meeting, 24 November 1983

[27] Ibid

[28] Ibid

[29] Walton, J., P. Beeson, and R. Bodley Scott, eds, *The Oxford Companion to Medicine Vol. 2 N–Z,* Oxford, Oxford University Press, 1986

[30] Extracts from the report of the CPSM Interim Inspection, 11–12 July 1983

[31] Ibid

Chapter 13
Upgrading and Course Development: 1984–1986

At the time of the interim inspection, the staffing position was looking promising and it appeared that the recruitment strategy was producing the anticipated results. However, there was no room for complacency as, within weeks, the school was returned to its precarious position when Jill Humphreys left on qualification as a teacher and Jean Webb returned to clinical work without completing the Certificate in Education course. Ann Neill was recruited for the 1983 Certificate in Education course at Dudley, funded by an arrangement with the West Midlands Regional Health Authority, who supported the fifteen-month course from regional funds.[1] She was lively and enthusiastic and, although she had not yet developed a high degree of specialisation in any one field, she had demonstrated a keen interest in each clinical area to which she had been deployed. She qualified as a teacher of physiotherapy in December 1984 having gained a distinction in coursework and remained on the staff until August 1987, when she married and left the area to take up a post at the Withington School of Physiotherapy. Jean Davies finally lost the battle to a long and painful illness in November 1984. Bobbie Goff and Jean Rogers, although officially retired, both returned to teaching to give generous support to staff and students through the school's continuing staffing crisis.

Phyl Fletcher-Cook and Cath Rose had numerically replaced Bobbie and Jean in January 1982 and March 1983 respectively. However, they had significantly less experience than the people they replaced and it was a great relief when Ken Stopani, a qualified, experienced teacher from Birmingham Royal Orthopaedic Hospital School of Physiotherapy, was appointed to the assistant principal post at Stoke-on-Trent in January 1984.[2] Oswestry-based staff had maintained the teaching schedule in

Stoke-on-Trent on a daily basis since Tony Fowler's departure three years before but they had little involvement with NSHA and the day-to-day operation of the Stoke-on-Trent branch of the school. Ken's appointment would re-establish the school presence in North Staffordshire and, it was hoped, would improve communication between the two Health Authorities.

Ken brought energy, experience and enthusiasm to his new post. Interested and innovative in all aspects of course delivery, he had gained particular knowledge of a broad range of assessment techniques that would subsequently be incorporated into the school's assessment programme. Together they made a good team; Ken's ideas combined with Marian's planning ability and attention to detail provided the foundation for subsequent successful course development.

Two new student teachers were recruited to the Certificate in Further Education course at Dudley in September 1984. They had come from areas where schools were established in higher education and openly stated their preferences to return to these environments on qualification for the higher salaries, improved conditions of service and the staffing levels that existed in higher education. Both gained a distinction in coursework, following Ann's achievement the previous year. Although the school lost Sue Hopkins in December 1985, it was fortunate to retain Margaret Grant as a staff member for a further year after which she returned to a lecturer's post in Glasgow.[3] Margaret contributed much to school life during her stay with her dedication to work and high standards of performance. She was a stimulating and perceptive teacher with a delightful sense of humour. She was driven to pursue the academic and clinical excellence so necessary for the profession, and enrolled on the MSc in Habilitation offered by Liverpool University. Glasgow Caledonian University continued to support her studies on her return and she completed the MSc in the minimal time. Nora Richards left the school on completion of her short-term contract and was almost immediately replaced by Jean Richards, a qualified, experienced teacher, who accepted a part-time contract of three days a week to boost the staffing levels to their highest point for some time. Jean's main responsibility was to support clinical teaching in Stoke-on-Trent.[4]

Marilyn Place was selected for the 1985 course. She had been, for a number of years, physiotherapist in charge of the intensive care unit in Shrewsbury and had made initial enquiries about teacher training a year before she was able to make the commitment to the course. She was concerned that the transfer from clinical work to the academic environment would render her ineffectual as a teacher once direct patient contact was lost. Marilyn's appointment was necessary to remedy the glaring shortfall of cardiovascular/respiratory expertise on the staff and her ultimate decision was awaited with a studied patience that belied Marian's inward panic lest the 'wrong' decision should be made.

When she finally came to the school, Marilyn's special abilities became immediately obvious. She challenged staff, school and students on every aspect of activity and attacked the course with an enthusiasm and vigour that left the establishment reeling. She followed three very successful student teachers all of whom had gained distinctions in coursework, but Marilyn surpassed this by also achieving the very rarely awarded distinction in teaching practice. She qualified and joined the staff in January 1987 and with subsequent studies for a master's degree in Education – also achieved with distinction – she was a singular and most valuable asset for the dramatic course development to be effected over the next few years. With strong leadership capabilities, highly developed interpersonal skills, the master's degree in Education and sound clinical expertise, she made an immediate significant contribution to course development, and by the early 1990s was leading the course development teams, taking responsibility specifically for the courses developed with Keele University.

The Education Committee was impressed by the level of student teacher recruitment but obviously had expected the newly qualified teachers to remain at the school. They were a little disconcerted to find that there was a continuing need to train yet more teachers. It was of little consolation to be informed that of the six student teachers who had qualified from the school since 1981, four were still actively teaching in West Midlands schools of physiotherapy. One was in Wolverhampton and three were at the ONSSP. One had worked in the school until her untimely death and one only had not continued in teaching.[5] After long discussion and hard negotiation, funding was approved to allow Shân Aguilar to undertake the 1986 Certificate in Education course.

However strong the teaching staff, no department can operate without adequate supportive office administration personnel and, for almost two decades, Janet Lymn had fulfilled this role during the tenure of three principals. Janet, who occupied the post of secretary then personal assistant to the principal, was the lynchpin about which all school activities revolved. She acted as liaison between the principal and staff, students, hospital administration, the Chartered Society of Physiotherapy and the Council for Professions Supplementary to Medicine. She also dealt with all the correspondence and administrative matters, rapidly coming to terms with Marian's minuscule writing and converting her scrawls into businesslike documents, lists or letters as required. Janet was always helpful, efficient and capable as she coped with the traumas of day-to-day activity with a reassuring cheerfulness and confidence that held the school together.

Her working conditions were terrible. She sat at a bench set at right angles to the door and had to look over her left shoulder to welcome visitors to the office. Her ancient typewriter had several idiosyncrasies, one of which was to punch holes in the letters o, a, b, d and e. Some improvements in her work environment were made before she retired by the purchase of a desk and word processor, and for her last years she was able to greet visitors by just raising her head rather than twisting her torso. Without her incredibly hard work and her ability to keep Marian conversant with the many internal and external procedures required, the school would have been in an even more parlous state. She acted as a buffer between the various factions, giving advice, support and encouragement, and provided many other services to the school.

Due to the constantly increasing pressures and Janet's planned departure in July 1986, permission was granted to appoint a part-time secretary to provide some overlap in the office. Once agreed, it took several months to arrange the finance and to complete the appointment procedures before Karen Bright was appointed.[6] She was confident and competent in most of the routine office procedures by the time Janet retired. Janet's departure left a potential gap in the organisation that was very concerning. However, the post attracted significant interest when advertised and Judy Bebb was among the applicants.[7]

She had already worked in the hospital for several years and was now looking for a post that was more challenging than the one she currently occupied. The stability of the workforce at the hospital determined that such posts did not arise frequently. Judy was young, bright, charming and very organised. Within days of appointment, she had streamlined the administrative functions within the school and had started to reorganise the office. It was a very happy solution to Janet's departure and Marian looked forward to many years of a pleasant and stimulating working relationship with Judy and hoped that she in turn would become more efficient in the administrative procedures that occupied such a large proportion of her time.

Following Jean Davies' untimely death in November 1984, her husband, Hugh, donated an annual prize in her memory. It was his wish that each student should have the opportunity of gaining this award, irrespective of individual academic ability. After much debate and information-seeking from other schools known to have similar prizes, it was decided that the award would be made each year to the student who excelled in the clinical field. Clinical educators were invited to nominate the candidates they thought most suitable to receive the award. It was recognised that students did not encounter every clinical educator, but, as the same number of placements were undertaken by each student during the course, it was considered that the distribution of votes would be fair and even.

It was fitting that the first presentation of the award should be in 1985, as the group of students about to qualify were those with whom Jean had spent her all too brief teaching career. She had taught movement studies during the first year of their course. Hugh Davies presented the prize to the outright winner, Lucy Oliver, who had been initially offered a place at the Bristol School of Physiotherapy. When the proposed intake to that school was suspended following the school's quinquennial CPSM inspection, Lucy applied to the ONSSP for a place to be taken up the following year.[8] Coincidentally, in 1986, one of the joint winners of the award was Jennifer Trott. She had also been offered a place on the suspended intake to the Bristol School and came to Oswestry in 1983. Lucy and Jennifer had been friends from their school days and, in the final year, Lucy had been head girl of the school and Jennifer her deputy.

The awards ceremony was now firmly established in the school's calendar and students invited as guests people who directly or indirectly had made a major contribution to their lives at the school. Miss Hollis, former principal of the Bradford Hospitals School of Physiotherapy, came in 1985. Author of the students' standard text on movement, she had trained Marian as a teacher and recruited Phyl Fletcher-Cook as student teacher immediately prior to her retirement. As Ken Stopani had gained his initial professional qualification from Bradford in the late '60s, there were three rather anxious members of staff on the platform on that occasion. It was more relaxed the following year when Mary Powell, the last matron of the hospital and author of a definitive textbook on orthopaedic nursing and physiotherapy, came to present the badges and awards. Mary's three sessions at Oswestry during her long and illustrious career started in 1936 when she trained as an orthopaedic nurse and physiotherapist; the second started in 1943 when she returned as assistant matron to the Gredington Children's Annexe. The third and final session was from 1962 to 1974 when she was first matron then principal nursing officer at the hospital.

Staff found the group who qualified in 1986 far more demanding than the two previous cohorts had been. As a group they were dedicated to their studies, occupying the new school library from the Christmas before their final examinations until these were completed. Despite the excessive shortages of teaching staff, an open-door policy had been introduced in 1981 and students were encouraged to seek tutorials as individuals or in small groups. There were many occasions during the second and third years of this cohort's passage when this decision was regretted. Two or three members of the year seemed continually to lie in wait for tutorial guidance that was far in excess of their needs, but they needed constant reassurance. Their examination results were very pleasing and, in the end, staff rewards were measured by their students' success.

Plans for the radical realignment of the course had been held in abeyance until success had been achieved in the July 1983 interim inspection. It was recognised that if the school was to produce an effective course with its traditionally low staffing levels, it had to be delivered more efficiently and, to this end, a block system was proposed for implementation in September 1984.[9]

The proposal was treated with extreme suspicion by clinical staff and administrators in both Health Authorities and also by the majority of the teaching staff. The only group who appeared to welcome the proposed change was the student body. Students, particularly those based at Stoke-on-Trent, had suffered most significantly by the continuing staff shortages. They could see the advantage of course teaching being focused on one site and felt a block system would give them a fairer deal. Teaching staff gave their reluctant support to the proposal when they were persuaded that, as a block system would obviate the need for the continued implementation of parallel course teaching at Stoke-on-Trent and Oswestry, they would have more time to participate in other educational activities with the students. Shropshire Health Authority accepted the proposal and was prepared to await implementation before making further comments, but North Staffordshire Health Authority was strongly opposed, expressing concerns that the loss of defined course teaching at Stoke-on-Trent would reduce the Authority's influence on the running of the school.

The implementation schedule had been planned in great detail to cause minimal disruption to students and staff. Marian was confident that, if her plan were followed precisely, the new block system would be phased in without problems arising. Each stage of the implementation required the circulation of detailed information/instruction packs to every member of staff prior to comprehensive meetings with students, in the school and at all hospital-based clinical sites.

The process was complicated by the lack of photocopying

facilities in the school. Janet Lymn spent many hours preparing the required packages of information using the hospital's photocopier located above the X-ray department. However, she had now been provided with a word processor which facilitated and improved the initial preparation of documents. All was progressing well until, in December 1983, Marian's health broke down and she required two months' recuperation. Despite having previously agreed the schedule, staff did not have the confidence to continue with implementation of the proposal and the final stages of the process had to await Marian's return to duty. Contrary to all predictions, the block system was finally introduced on schedule with no unforeseen problems arising and with immediate benefits for staff and students.

Ken Stopani, employed by North Staffordshire Health Authority from January 1984, attended his first Education Committee meeting in February while Marian was still on sick leave. He reported to this meeting that students based at Stoke-on-Trent felt very isolated from the mainstream of the school although they recognised that their living and teaching accommodation had improved substantially.[10] They still had no easy access to relevant study facilities despite the arrangements made for them at Haywood Hospital. The reason for this was that the school library was totally inadequate with a low supply of out-of-date textbooks. This was inappropriate as much of their learning was, of necessity, by self-directed study. There were also frequent problems with transport to the main hospital sites for their clinical education. Clinical staff who had always been very supportive were under great pressure due to their inadequate staffing levels and found their additional defined responsibilities towards students hard to maintain.

It had become progressively more difficult to continue with the upgrading programme required by the CPSM; however, Ken Stopani's appointment to North Staffordshire facilitated improvements in that section of the school. A budget for the school was identified and approximately £10,000 allocated by the Health Authority for new equipment and books at Stoke-on-Trent. Significant monies were also approved for the upgrading of the physiotherapy department at City General Hospital.[11]

1984 was an important year in the history of the Oswestry and North Staffordshire School of Physiotherapy as it marked the seventy-fifth anniversary of the founding of the massage school at Baschurch. The event was marked by the Old Oswestrian Physiotherapists Association at their annual meeting in May when a special cake to celebrate the event was cut by Greta Anderson, the most distant surviving principal, supported by Wyn Cannell and Marian Tidswell. The school was also entered in the Lichfield Diocesan Prayer Diary in June, with prayers for continued success in its chosen tasks.

Staff who had coped magnificently during the years of excessive staff shortages considered ruefully that they had neither the resources nor energy to comply with the ultimate CSP challenge presented during 1984. The CSP had found it increasingly difficult to maintain the national professional entrance examination for physiotherapy owing to the high costs of implementation and the small number of candidates involved. The system was expensive to operate and the number of candidates for which it catered was considered too small for statistical educational validity. They determined they could not continue despite an annual candidate pool of approximately 1,000 and drawing on the experience and expertise of approximately 250 teachers. The CSP determined that it would cease the national examination from the 1989 intake and by that time all schools wishing to continue to qualify physiotherapists would have to have produced validated internally assessed courses for approximately forty candidates annually, supported by an average of six staff.

The CSP had been encouraging schools to internalise their courses for a number of years, but, by 1984, only those that had already transferred to higher education bases had achieved this development. These schools freely admitted that, despite being fully staffed, internalisation would have been impossible without significant assistance from the experienced, dedicated examination departments of their hosting institutions. Owing to the timing of the cessation of the national examinations, although CSP requested implementation of new courses by 1986, the last date for them to start was autumn 1989. A further decision taken in

1985 separated qualification and membership that enabled the CSP Licence to Practice to be awarded to courses approved by the CPSM/CSP. Provided all the required elements of the CSP curriculum were incorporated, these courses could be awarded degrees by academic institutions.[12] Separation of qualification and membership appeared at the time to be a minor change but, actually, it was most significant, presenting every school with the opportunity and means to develop graduate courses.

When the CSP announced the discontinuance of the national examination system, the school's extreme vulnerability was again highlighted to the Education Committee and the two Health Authorities.[13] The school was still struggling to maintain course teaching with insufficient manpower to consider implementation of a valid assessment programme. However, if the instruction were not complied with, the school would accept its last cohort in 1988. The new courses were to be validated by the CPSM and CSP prior to implementation by school staff and would be monitored by CSP-appointed external examiners. The CSP had given five years' warning prior to implementation of the change – adequate time for individual schools to determine their future.

At the time of the announcement, Marian was the only CSP examiner in the school and teaching staff levels were so low that all energies were necessarily directed towards course maintenance rather than development. However, Ken Stopani had been appointed to the staff in January 1984 and, although a qualified teacher for more than five years, he had not yet applied to be an examiner. This situation was remedied immediately, doubling the school's complement of CSP-approved examiners. Phyl Fletcher-Cook was admitted to the Part 1 panel of examiners in 1985 and Jean Richards on her arrival at the school applied for the Part 2 panel.

The Education Committee was asked to identify the development route to be taken by the school. The urgency of the situation was stressed to avoid losing time in the pursuit of inappropriate or invalid development proposals.[14] Unfortunately, the mechanism for this level of decision-making did not exist within the Education Committee as it had no direct contact with the District Management Teams in either Health Authority.

These major communication problems were restricting all aspects of the school's progress and had been recognised by the CPSM interim inspection report.[15]

This communication issue was the only recommendation still outstanding from the 1983 CPSM inspection report and progress was finally to be made.[16] An outstanding issue from the 1981 CPSM inspection report was definition of the principal's position in the North Staffordshire Health Authority, as her contract of employment was Shropshire-based. This also now required urgent consideration if the school was to remain viable. After significant discussion in both Health Authorities it was decided that management arrangements in North Staffordshire Health Authority should mirror those already existing in Shropshire. It was confirmed that as the principal was accountable to Dr Moore, the district medical officer in SHA, in NSHA she would be accountable to Mr Fletcher, the district administrator.[17]

The next stage was to establish an Executive Committee with the ability to make significant decisions concerning the school's future and the authority to command the use of any resources required to implement their decisions. The committee would meet annually, or as required, and would be attended by the treasurer from each HA, Dr Moore and Mr Fletcher, the principal's defined managers in each HA, the principal and the secretary of the School Education Committee. The Executive Committee would coordinate the support of the school by the two separate authorities and make decisions on future policy. It was to discuss the funding arrangements for the school, determine annual budgets and agree the financial apportionment of costs between the two Health Authorities. Finally, it was to encourage educational development of the school in line with national policies of the professional and statutory bodies.[18] The proposals, when submitted to the District Management Teams in Shropshire and North Staffordshire Health Authorities, were approved and the Executive Committee was established.

Once the CSP decision to cease the national examination system was announced, it was recognised all staff would require additional skills and knowledge to support their enhanced role in future course development and implementation. Ken identified a location that provided training in a variety of course development activities. The courses had been established for medical personnel, but it was ascertained that physiotherapists would be welcome to attend. Having the training budget monies available, Marian was able to arrange staff attendance on several of the courses offered and staff learned the rudiments of course planning, curriculum design and a range of assessment methods including Objective Structured Clinical Examinations.

The Objective Structured Clinical Examination (OSCE) and its partner, the Objective Structured Practical Examination (OSPE), enabled a precise objective marking system in the assessment of clinical and practical skills. They ensured that examinations in these areas could be marked with the same rigour as written examinations and eliminated the subjective element that had previously been apparent. Staff worked enthusiastically to produce a bank of tasks to be performed and immediately introduced these forms of examination to the internal assessment programme of the school. Teaching staff ran workshops to train clinical supervisors in this system of examination. Also, following a presentation to a joint conference of physiotherapy teachers and managers in July 1985, the school was asked to present a three-day workshop for the Chartered Society of Physiotherapy, implemented at Stoke-on-Trent in November 1986 and attended by twenty-four teachers from different schools. School staff presented the theoretical component of the workshop and students on secondment to Stoke-on-Trent acted as models for practical sessions, runners and general hosts to the visitors.

In order to develop and implement a fully internalised course the immediate appointment of a minimum of three additional experienced teachers, already enrolled as CSP Part 1 and/or Part 2 Examiners, was required. Alternatively, the school could develop a degree course in collaboration with an appropriate institution sited in the higher education environment. By following this route, the examination department of the host institution would assist staff to develop and evaluate the assessment system, reducing the requirement for additional staff.

The first major task for the newly constituted Executive Committee was to decide the optimum course development route to be followed by the school and to brief the two MDTs so that the ultimate decision could be made. Both proposals were totally unrealistic as the two Health Authorities had consistently refused to increase teaching establishments or to implement the degree course developed with Chester College, mainly on financial grounds. The only realistic choice appeared to be to allow the school to close, but this was also unacceptable given the level of support and the efforts already made by all concerned to avert the proposed closure in 1983.

A possible solution to the problem was presented in July 1984 when the school of Physical Education and Recreation (SPEAR), a component department of Liverpool University, approached the school with a proposal for the development of a degree in physiotherapy and movement science.[19] This development would alleviate the insurmountable staffing problems associated with internalisation by providing access to the established and proven expertise of the university's examination department as well as providing course qualifiers with graduate entry to the profession. As five schools of physiotherapy already ran validated degree programmes incorporating the CSP Licence to Practice, this proposal was in line with current thinking and the school sought approval from the CSP for the proposed development. CSP encouraged the proposal and detailed discussions on course arrangements were instituted. Liverpool University approved the course development in principle and proposed 1986 as the target date for implementation of the course.

Ken Stopani, Marian Tidswell and Dr Brodie prepared the course documentation required, assisted by Phillip Holbourn, who was employed by the school and funded against staff vacancies. He had excellent skills in documentation and prepared critical path analyses of all essential physiotherapy components of the course, demonstrating clearly the academic route for undergraduates to follow in the acquisition of clinical competence. It was to the school's advantage that he was not a physiotherapist as he reviewed all professional and academic requirements dispassionately and presented subsequent information in a clearly understood format without professional bias. This was considered necessary in order to satisfy the varied expertise of the subsequent reviewers of the course and its documentation.

As this extra work was progressing in the school, an appraisal of the probable costs of implementation of the proposed course in collaboration with SPEAR was made by Shropshire Health Authority and presented to the Executive Committee.[20] Stoke-on-Trent representatives on the committee initially queried why SPEAR had been chosen without prior consultation with Staffordshire-based institutions. They were assured that the approach had been made by SPEAR, not the school, and were reminded of the CSP's decision to cease national examinations. The unsatisfactory outcome of the 1982 discussions to the course prepared with Chester College in response to a direct instruction contained in the 1981 CPSM inspection report was also noted. Further procrastination was not possible if the school was to continue after 1989.

The Executive Committee proposed negotiation of reduction of the costs of course implementation with Liverpool University as they had been estimated to be three times the figures quoted by Chester two years before. Meantime, NSHA had negotiated an advantageous position with regard to the apportionment of additional costs to be incurred by the two Health Authorities irrespective of the development ultimately pursued. They agreed to present the SPEAR proposal to the NSHA for approval.[21] Unfortunately, this was not effected and by May 1985, although SHA had granted approval for the course development some months earlier, North Staffordshire had not as yet presented the proposal to the MDT. Course organisers, the school and SPEAR were concerned that, with the delays in the decision-making process, an October 1986 start to the proposed course was now impossible and it was already looking doubtful that a course could be prepared and validated in time for 1987.[22]

At a joint meeting between representatives of the two funding Health Authorities held two months later, the discussions held originally by the school Education Committee were readdressed. All aspects of the debate already conducted in several forums had another airing. By the end of the meeting, participants agreed to recommend to North Staffordshire's MDT that a link with Liverpool University be agreed in principle provided the school encouraged further local recruitment of its student population, in line with recruitment patterns in radiography. If the MDT supported the recommendation, then, following the October meeting of the Health Authority, officers from North Staffordshire would join in any discussions with SPEAR as there was a declared interest to develop physiotherapy education on a truly joint basis.[23]

Course development continued and documentation was presented to Liverpool University for initial validation prior to submission to the CPSM/CSP Joint Submissions Committee. This 'validation event' occurred in June 1986. At this meeting, school representatives watched with horror as the course, so carefully planned, was deconstructed by the university professors present. They appeared to disregard the physiotherapy professional requirements and apportioned the proposed additional revenues agreed by the Health Authorities between their departments with little if any consideration of the course proposal. Marian was particularly concerned that, if the revised proposal were to be accepted, the course as approved would commit the funding Health Authorities to considerable expenditure without providing graduates the essential licence to practise physiotherapy. She had no option other than to recommend discontinuance of the discussions and accept with mounting concern that the two years spent on negotiation of the degree had been wasted; the school was no further forward in its search for a viable future than it had been in 1984.

The effects of the 1982 NHS reorganisation were now devolving downwards and the RJAH was identified as the main hospital in the new northern unit of Shropshire Health Authority. Jeff Silk, after serving a number of years as sector administrator at the Robert Jones and Agnes Hunt Orthopaedic Hospital, secured employment in another Health Authority following a year's secondment to an alternative post in SHA.[24] On his return to the hospital, Jeff attended only two meetings of the Education Committee. David Blaxland was appointed locum tenens during Jeff's initial absence.

Jeff's imminent departure had a devastating effect on the school's morale as he had given consistent support and encouragement to staff through a very difficult time. A diplomatic yet forceful negotiator, he inspired confidence in both staff and students. Sensitive to individual needs, fully conversant with the different requirements of the professional and statutory bodies, he was very knowledgeable about the complexities of physiotherapy education. It is doubtful if the school could have survived the aftermath of the 1981 CPSM inspection without this blend of knowledge and experience assisting the new principal through her first years of tenure of the post.

Jeff's replacement was Gordon Braid, the first appointed unit general manager (UGM) of the northern unit of Shropshire Health Authority. At the same time, Dr Moore, Marian's line manager in Shropshire Health Authority, retired and was replaced by Martin Beardwell, director of personnel in SHA. At a stroke, the management team that had supported the school in Shropshire so effectively since 1981 was demolished and replaced by people with personal agendas to satisfy the demands of the latest NHS reorganisation rather than the needs of the school.

The two school bases were now located in units of the parent Health Authorities. North Staffordshire Health Authority was characterised by a strong management team and supportive environment where all levels of authority and accountability were clearly defined. The school moved easily from the previous management system to the new one in North Staffordshire and a relaxed working relationship was developed with the new unit manager, Tony Heywood. Shropshire Health Authority, by contrast, appeared to have indecisive district management backed by aggressive unit management, which was to be problematical for the school over the next few years.

For reasons of efficiency and effectiveness, some professions, including physiotherapy, had developed district-wide services managed by discipline-specific functional managers who had responsibility for all personnel and financial management of their individual clinical services. This had proved an effective way to improve service delivery, particularly for patients and staff dependent on small, scattered hospitals or based in the community. This arrangement was, however, against the principles of unit management that assumed unit control of all clinical services provided by the hospital. During the first few months of unit management in Shropshire, the effective district-wide services were dismantled with each treatment base receiving its apportioned share of the overall budget according to the level of the services provided. District therapists lost their management role and reverted to being advisors with no management brief. The quality of service received by patients in the smaller hospitals deteriorated.

The UGM considered the school occupied an unwarranted position of privilege within the Authority and, after having successfully dismantled district-based clinical services, declared his intent to 'unitise' the school to bring it into line with other hospital departments. Successful management of the school was incompatible with the principles of unit control owing to the CPSM/CSP requirement for all schools to be managed at district level that, in this case, spanned responsibility across the two Health Authorities. This was to prove to be an insurmountable problem.

The only area of the school's responsibility over which the UGM had undisputed control was the accommodation based in 'his' unit and this was attacked with vigour. There were still some minor alterations to be completed in the school before the 1986 CPSM/CSP inspection and, as the monies originally allocated had been timed out and further development monies were not forthcoming, the essential required funds were raised by using underspends on the school budget. The school funded the development of two seminar rooms that were completed prior to the routine quinquennial inspection on the 5 and 6 October 1986 with the confidence that all items raised by the two previous reports had now been completed satisfactorily and student and staff facilities matched professional norms.

This euphoria was short-lived as, on 15 October, the UGM demanded immediate clearance of the seminar rooms as they were required for use as the hospital transport office. He stated that it was only his consideration for the school that had allowed retention of the rooms until after the CPSM inspection. Now that was over, relocation of the transport office could be effected. Replacement rooms were promised by 1 January 1997, but despite the school raising sufficient money year on year from underspends on the school budget to replace them, they were not reinstated for another three years. Students and staff made frequent representation to unit management, but their entreaties met with negative responses and each year the money the school had saved was used by the Unit to offset its deficit or fund some small development in another department. Student residential accommodation was also disrupted by the displacement of finalist students from the study block built specifically for them in the late 1960s. They were relocated in the main Nurses' Home, in rooms scattered throughout the building that were too small to accommodate a desk. Second-year students were also subjected to unnecessary room changes.

Following rebuilding of the hospital after the 1948 fire, the administration office suite had occupied rooms located midway along the main corridor directly opposite the original hospital entrance between Ercall Ward and Wrekin Ward. This was no longer considered satisfactory and the UGM sought a new venue. First-year physiotherapy students occupied study bedrooms and a sitting room in the end wing of the Nurses' Home adjacent to the new hospital entrance. The wing could be isolated from the hurly-burly of the home's life, providing solitude and peace to study. This was the location the UGM selected for his new suite of offices. Protest was ineffectual as each contact or comment made about student disruption appeared to stimulate further activity. It appeared to be the UGM's intention to make their lives as difficult as possible and to demonstrate to the maximum the extent of his influence on the school's activities. He considered students were ill-disciplined and out of control, and made many unjust and unsubstantiated complaints about their perceived behavioural aberrations. On each occasion he demanded extreme measures be taken against the named students allegedly concerned. This was not required as the allegations were never substantiated.

The initial five-year plan for the school had been totally implemented by the end of 1986. Staff numbers were steadily increasing, accommodation and equipment upgrades had been completed and course development was under way. There was a new concern about the activities of the Regional Training Councils in relation to all aspects of professional education, and the school entered 1987 with some trepidation.

Notes

[1] Extracts from the minutes of the ONSSP Education Committee meeting, 19 May 1983

[2] Extracts from the minutes of the ONSSP Education Committee meeting, 15 February 1984

[3] Extracts from the minutes of the ONSSP Education Committee meeting, 23 September 1986

[4] Extracts from the minutes of the ONSSP Education Committee meeting, 21 January 1985

[5] Ibid

[6] Extracts from the minutes of the ONSSP Education Committee meeting, 21 May 1985

[7] Extracts from the minutes of the ONSSP Education Committee meeting, 6 May 1986

[8] Extracts from the minutes of the ONSSP Education Committee meeting, 24 September 1985

[9] Extracts from the report of the CPSM Interim Inspection, 11–12 July 1983

[10] Extracts from the minutes of the ONSSP Education Committee meeting, 15 February 1984

[11] Extracts from the minutes of the ONSSP Education Committee meeting, 16 May 1984

[12] Chartered Society of Physiotherapy, '100 years 1894–1994', *Physiotherapy* vol. 80 issue A, 1994

[13] Extracts from the minutes of the ONSSP Education Committee meeting, 15 August 1984

[14] Ibid

[15] Extracts from the report of the CPSM Interim Inspection, 11–12 July 1983

[16] Extracts from the minutes of the ONSSP Education Committee meeting, 16 May 1984

[17] Ibid

[18] Ibid

[19] Extracts from the minutes of the ONSSP Education Committee meeting, 15 August 1984

[20] Extracts from the minutes of the ONSSP Executive Education Committee meeting, 25 October 1984

[21] Extracts from the minutes of the ONSSP Education Committee meeting, 28 November 1984

[22] Extracts from the minutes of the ONSSP Education Committee meeting, 21 May 1985

[23] Extracts from notes of a joint meeting between representatives of North Staffordshire and Shropshire Health Authorities, 8 July 1985

[24] Extracts from the minutes of the ONSSP Education Committee meeting, 16 May 1984

Chapter 14
Regional Training Council Activity: 1987

Regional Training Councils (RTCs) were established in the early 1980s primarily to ensure the most efficient use of resources. Information gained from the professions covered by the councils was to be used for manpower planning and the development of post-registration courses for qualified staff. The West Midlands region, covering twenty-two Health Authorities from Coventry to the Welsh Borders, established a Regional Training Council (RTC) with membership of district general managers, personnel officers and nursing representatives to review regional facilities for post-registration education. The RTC then established Staff Development Groups (SDGs) to consider manpower planning in, and post-registration development of, other individual professional groups. Exclusion of staff concerned with pre-registration education from direct membership of the SDG necessitated co-option on to additional subcommittees to report relevant information to the parent committee. Through this mechanism, recommendations were implemented to increase occupational therapy and chiropody training and to reduce radiography training in the region.

One of the SDGs was devoted to physiotherapy and, although it was concerned initially with post-registration education opportunities for the profession, it subsequently expanded its remit to cover pre-registration education as an aspect of manpower planning. To facilitate communication between the clinical and educational branches of the service, the Physiotherapy Evaluation Group (PEG) was established to give advice on educational matters. Two principals from the region were elected on behalf of the five schools of physiotherapy to liaise with the PEG. These were Marian Tidswell and Doreen Caney. Marian, principal of the ONSSP, was an elected member of the CSP

Council and Doreen, principal of the Queen Elizabeth School of Physiotherapy, Birmingham, was an elected physiotherapy board member of the CPSM. They were invited to prepare a report identifying the existing arrangements for, and the status of, physiotherapy education in the West Midlands region. This was presented to the PEG in December 1985, only to be rejected by the chairman of the SDG on the grounds that it identified a national perspective on physiotherapy education and the SDG was concerned only with the regional view. The chairman of the SDG and senior training officer of WMRHA subsequently rewrote the report with regional emphasis and incorporated the revised information into the SDG report on the region's manpower needs for publication by the WMRHA in 1986.

The final draft of this report was presented in strict confidence to the five principals and their line managers in February 1986 and contained a paragraph recommending that the ONSSP should be closed in September of that year. The basis for this action was that the school had not as yet gained approval from the CPSM/CSP for an internally assessed course. Naturally there were strong objections to the inclusion of the recommendation as the report's declared intentions had been to identify the existing provision of physiotherapy education; questions concerning future development of courses had not been requested in the original remit. It was also questioned if the SDG had the authority to recommend closure of a school that met fully the statutory and professional requirements determined by the Council for Professions Supplementary to Medicine and the Chartered Society of Physiotherapy.

The offending paragraph was removed and all the people attending the meeting agreed to maintain total confidentiality about the contents and discussions relating to the draft. They were assured that they were the only people other than the authors to have seen it; however, there had been a wider circulation and other readers were not bound by any confidentiality agreement. The school became aware of this when a candidate who had applied, been interviewed and offered a place at the ONSSP for the September 1986 intake later withdrew her application. On investigating the situation, the school was informed by the applicant's headmaster that he had advised his pupil to withdraw from the ONSSP and apply to another school to guarantee continuity of her course. He had been informed by an 'unimpeachable source' at CSP headquarters that the ONSSP was to close. The following year, the school received no applications for the scheduled 1987 intake and on enquiry discovered that it had been omitted from the CSP list of approved schools. Action taken on the content of the final draft of the report had not been corrected when the definitive document was published four months later. This resulted in a delay in selection of this cohort and the number of potential students recruited for the 1987 intake was less than in previous years, with only twenty provisional places being offered.

The WMRHA SDG report was produced in June 1986.[1] It identified the need to review the existing provision of physiotherapy pre-registration education in the West Midlands and relate it specifically to projected regional manpower needs. Significant reductions in training capacity were proposed and a study of the feasibility of amalgamating, closing or rationalising the five schools in the region to reduce the existing annual intake of 140 students to the calculated projected regional requirement of seventy new qualifiers per annum was recommended.

A new PEG was formed with a WMRHA-based district general manager (DGM) appointed chairman. The principals previously elected to report to the PEG were invited to join the new group, but declined, identifying that all five schools should be represented or none at all to allow unbiased presentation of each school's interest. Full representation of the schools was naturally rejected and the compromise solution was to appoint an independent principal from a school of physiotherapy located in another region. Incidentally, this independent member principal was later criticised severely by the chairman of the PEG for emphasising the national perspective on physiotherapy education. In addition to this independent principal, the group's membership comprised three district physiotherapists and the WMRHA assistant training manager. The Group's remit was to:

- initiate an early evaluation of the effectiveness of the pilot scheme at Coventry (Lanchester) Polytechnic

- implement a feasibility study to assess the viability of integration of schools of physiotherapy into higher education establishments and consider the amalgamation of NHS schools within the West Midlands RHA.

The mechanism for the conduct of the feasibility study was determined and presented to the principals and their line managers at a meeting in Birmingham in March 1987. The UGM northern unit SHA was nominated to represent and support the school as neither of the principals' line managers were available to attend the meeting. The next few months were occupied by completion of many forms and lists of requested information as the PEG planned visits to the five schools of the region. As her line managers had been unable to attend the initial briefing, the principal insisted that they each scrutinised the initial documentation she prepared before submission to the PEG to ensure both Health Authorities were in total agreement with the information presented by the school. They both commented that the submission was of a professional standard and proposed no alteration to either the content or the manner of presentation of the information.

The PEG inspection team initially expressed reluctance to visit the two sections of the ONSSP as visits to the other schools had been completed in a half day. However, common sense prevailed and both school bases received the same level of attention from the team on 28 April 1987. Members of the team asked many questions of the people they met and although some of these questions appeared to be quite obscure, the visitors were courteous and polite and appeared to be satisfied with the content of their visits. Following the visit, students commented that many of the questions they had been asked were directed towards their perceptions of the conditions under which they studied rather than the quality of the education received. It disconcerted staff to be asked to nominate a school within the region to which they would transfer in the event of the closure of their own establishment. The visits were comprehensive and the report was awaited with confidence, secure in the knowledge that the school had been presented in a positive and accurate manner. Early in June

1987 further information was requested and submitted concerning the progress with plans for course development.

Rumours concerning the school's future started to circulate early in June. Clinicians from other disciplines within the RJAH questioned school staff about the timing and reasons for the school's impending closure. On contact with the principal's line manager in Shrewsbury to request confirmation or denial of the accuracy of the rumour, the school was informed in confidence that 'a recommendation of unknown content' was to be put to a meeting of the PEG on 19 June. This might be accepted or rejected at a later meeting and if accepted would take further time to implement. Over the next few weeks the school was bombarded with requests for further information. These came mainly from a range of interested parties external to the hospital and finally, on 25 June 1987, hospital engineers appeared during teaching hours to measure up the classrooms preparatory to conversion of the rooms to offices. Mr Beardwell, the principal's line manager, met with the teaching staff on 17 June to inform them, in confidence, that a recommendation to suspend the 1987 intake to the school was to be presented to the RTC the following day. It is considered that school staff respected this confidence. The UGM was also been informed in confidence of the proposed recommendation.

The schedule for dissemination of information was that the report was finalised at a meeting of the PEG on Friday, 19 June 1987 prior to ratification by the RTC on 24 June. The contents of the report, the PEG interim statement, were disclosed finally on Friday, 26 June 1987 to a joint meeting of members of the group, principals of the five schools and their line managers.[2] Arrangements for this meeting were made with maximum confidentiality, initially by telephone and later confirmed by letter. No agenda was circulated and it was reinforced that the contents of the report to be presented at the meeting were as yet unknown and highly confidential. This was rather insulting in view of the leaks that had already occurred and the rumours that had been circulating freely throughout the region for the past few weeks.

The timing of the report's publication was excellent. Students had completed their examinations and awaited the results. Shân

Aguilar was scheduled to return to the school in September on completion of the college-based component of her teacher-training course and Jane Holmes had been accepted for the September 1987 course.

The recommendations presented to the meeting were as follows:

1. An embargo to be placed on admittance to ONSSP in 1987 and the twenty students already offered a place at the school to be redirected to alternative schools in the West Midlands.
2. Recruitment and selection for the 1988 ONSSP student intake to be suspended.
3. The level of student intake within the West Midlands Region in 1987 and 1988 to be maintained with the full CPSM approved intake of 148 distributed across four schools instead of five.
4. Clinical placements developed by the ONSSP to be protected and made available to other schools in the region.
5. Final decision/agreements to be concluded between principals of schools and higher education establishments only with the prior written approval of the RTC.
6. Funds allocated by the Shropshire and North Staffordshire Health Authorities for support of the 1987 intake at the ONSSP to be used to finance the transfer of that intake to other schools and staff vacancy funds also to be used to facilitate that transfer.[3]

It was further proposed that Shân Aguilar should transfer to the Wolverhampton school to complete her course and Jane Holmes, the student teacher approved and accepted by the ONSSP, would transfer to Wolverhampton for the September 1987 course. It appeared that the first part of the PEG's published remit, with regard to the course run by the Coventry school, had been ignored and the group had concentrated exclusively on the rationalisation of physiotherapy education provision in the region.

Immediate individual responses to the content of the statement were mixed. Helen Atkinson, principal of the Coventry school, supported Marian Tidswell's contention that there was no sound basis for the recommendation to close the ONSSP. NSHA representatives expressed concern about the proposed closure, but were happy to offer the school's clinical placements to the other schools in the region. SHA representatives accepted their commitment to continue to support students currently in training if they transferred to other schools to complete their studies. They were, however, significantly dismayed to discover that they were expected to support students accepted for the 1987 intake although these students would, in all probability, not attend the ONSSP. Also, as the predicted regional manpower requirement had been increased from the seventy of the previous report[4] to 148, twenty-eight of those potential students were identified as SHA's allocated financial responsibility. This was not welcome news as, for the previous seven years, they had funded only twenty bursary places despite the approved intake of the school having been increased from twenty to twenty-four in 1983 and from twenty-four to twenty-eight by the October 1986 CPSM/CSP inspection teams.

Two members of the PEG agreed to attend the Oswestry base of the school on Tuesday, 30 June to impart the news directly to staff, students and the school policy committee. Before the meeting closed all in attendance agreed to maintain total confidentiality about the recommendations contained in the report until after this date. Despite these promises, ONSSP staff were apprised of the detail of the day's proceedings by colleagues from other schools before the Shropshire contingent had returned to base.

The chairman of the PEG wrote to the principal on 29 June to say that the 'Group had considered the points raised by her and her line manager at the meeting but commented that their representations warranted no amendment to the interim statement'.[5] The letter was copied to the personnel from the other schools attendant at the meeting the previous Friday and was received by the ONSSP on 3 July, after the PEG representatives had imparted their news.

At separate meetings on 30 June, the PEG representatives met with teaching staff, students, John Stockbridge (Chairman of the ONSSP policy committee) and Ron Jones (deputising for Martin Beardwell). Students and staff asked many pertinent questions, to which they received no valid responses, merely a dogmatic reiteration of the proposals. They were all frustrated by the lack of realistic justification for the decisions taken.

Now that the report was officially in the public domain, an active campaign was mounted to challenge the recommendations. Newspaper, radio and television coverage was quite extensive. The local population was generous in its support as was the RJAH Medical Advisory Committee, the Institute of Orthopaedics and other departments from the hospital. Chris Bond, the CSP student officer, gave unstinting support and encouragement to the students, arranging for them to meet with the CSP director of education, physiotherapy education advisor and the principal to mount a campaign against the proposals. Students were interviewed on radio, raised a national petition that gained thousands of signatures and demonstrated with dignity outside the building in which a Regional Health Authority meeting was being conducted. The only direct contact between the RHA and the school occurred when representatives from this demonstration were invited to meet with the chairman of the RHA, who subsequently praised them for the manner in which they had stated their case and the clarity of their arguments.

The principal attended many meetings in London and throughout the West Midlands, asking questions, seeking answers, refuting the PEG's statements and desperately seeking the means to overturn the recommendations to restore the status quo. Members of staff were devastated by the news and morale was very low. The longer the uncertainty persisted, the less likely the school would be to recover from this assault and staff soon came to realise that, unless the decisions were reversed very quickly, they would not be in a position to cope with the September intake, regardless of their initial enthusiasm.

A meeting between the RTC, CSP and CPSM was held in Birmingham on 8 July and lasted for many hours. The outcome was that the CSP wrote to the RHA objecting to the decisions taken and the recommendations contained in the interim statement. This had the effect of retarding the proposed ratification of the report by the RTC that had been scheduled for 15 July. It was further proposed that urgent meetings should take place between the teaching staffs of the ONSSP and the Wolverhampton school to determine if there was any acceptable basis on which the two schools could merge. This meeting was held at Stowe House, Lichfield, on 15 July when staff from the two schools spent several hours with syllabi, teaching and clinical education schedules attempting to mesh the courses, to little effect. ONSSP staff left the meeting even more depressed as it determined that the schools were unable, at that time, to cooperate to determine a strategy that would lead to eventual amalgamation of the two courses. ONSSP staff were not prepared to see their successful course totally annihilated and Wolverhampton staff were unable to compromise the course with internalised assessment procedures they had already developed to accommodate an enforced merger. The failure to agree a strategy for amalgamation was communicated to Phil Mogg, the regional training officer at the subsequent meeting attended by all staff of the two schools, the education officer and director of education of the CSP. It was another long and arduous meeting that ended in a heated exchange between the principal of the ONSSP and the regional training officer. Finally, Mr Mogg indicated that if CSP would give approval for the ONSSP to accept the 1987 cohort, the RTC would raise no objections.

An emergency meeting of the school policy committee was convened for 27 July, when the interim statement was discussed at length, action already taken identified and plans for the future proposed. The principal's line managers reported the responses sent by their respective Health Authorities to the regional personnel manager and regional training officer stating 'that support could not be given for the interim statement in the absence of any reasoned argument to support the recommendations'.[6] Mr Beardwell also reported the outcome of the meeting with Wolverhampton staff when it had become obvious that a merger of the two schools was not a practical proposition at that time.

He reported that, following that meeting, ONSSP teaching

staff had determined they wished to produce a document for submission to the CSP/CPSM with proposals for an internalised course to refute another of the PEG's criticisms of the school. It was again identified, as on previous occasions, that such a course could not readily be implemented without an increase in the teaching establishment, although the documentation could be produced at an early stage.[7] NSHA was concerned about the major policy change in the school's proposed course development and after discussion it was determined that degree negotiations should continue alongside the proposals for internalisation until such time as a final decision had to be made.

In subsequent representation to the CSP, active support for the school was demanded as it met all statutory and professional requirements, confirmed by the October 1986 CPSM/CSP inspection report. The region's proposals not only negated that report, but also jeopardised the status of the schools to which it had been proposed to relocate ONSSP students as the additional numbers on their courses would cause each school to exceed its approved annual intake. Staff/student ratios would be upset and it was possible that school facilities would not meet CPSM/CSP approval for the increased student populations. These points, together with all other representations, were finally successful in achieving the overturn of the interim statement by the end of July. The ONSSP 1987 cohort was notified and preparations made for their arrival. When these students came to take Part 1 in June 1988, they achieved a 100 per cent pass in the examination, indicating they had come to terms with the uncertainty of the location of their studies produced by the interim statement.

The RTC published its definitive report[8] in December 1987. The publication date was again fortuitous as, being immediately before the Christmas break, it presented the opportunity to consider the contents fully while students were on leave. Reasoned arguments were presented to support the recommendations made and it was a far more professional presentation than the interim statement had been. However, the inaccuracies and prejudices that had devalued the earlier attempt to introduce radical change in the pattern of physiotherapy education provision across the region were repeated and augmented in the new report. Also, around the time of the report's publication, discussions were under way between the profession and the government that would, if successful, alter the basis of the funding of physiotherapy pre-registration education.[9] It was considered therefore that many of the proposals presented in the report were either inappropriate and/or presented at the wrong time.

The first recommendation was that the West Midland Region should train physiotherapists exclusively to meet service and manpower needs taking account of the natural wastage identified in its strategic plan.[10] To this end, the report recommended an annual intake of 120 students across the region, a reduction of twenty-eight from the numbers identified by the interim statement published less than six months earlier. It was proposed also that preference should be given to the recruitment of applicants living within the region's boundaries. This was in direct conflict with information submitted by the schools who had already identified to the PEG that students who came to the region to train were far more likely to remain on qualification than those recruited from within regional boundaries.

Three of the West Midland schools were described as being sited in modern, purpose-built premises.[11] These establishments were described as being well-equipped and regional representatives considered they were each capable of accommodating an annual intake of forty students. It was proposed that they should be encouraged to recruit to this target number. On acceptance of the report, the region's future education provision should concentrate on these three sites and provided an explanation for the proposed reduction in student numbers. Accommodation based on 'split sites' at the ONSSP and Coventry school was described as unsatisfactory. It was proposed that Coventry should become the region's post-registration education centre and development of a top-up degree in rehabilitation for regionally based physiotherapists was proposed. As it was now surplus to the initial training requirements, the ONSSP was to close.[12]

It was also proposed that the clinical placements for the programmes run by the five schools should be confined to the region. All DHAs should be encouraged to establish and support clinical education placements to maximise exposure to the range of clinical experience available across the region.[13] Two schools, the ONSSP and Queen Elizabeth School, Birmingham, already complied with this recommendation. The ONSSP had long recognised that a major benefit to the school was the wealth of appropriate pre-qualification clinical education opportunities available within the two funding Health Authorities. The high-quality clinical education programme developed by the school was, at that time, implemented totally within NSHA and SHA geographical boundaries. The Queen Elizabeth school had a wider distribution of placements, but all were contained within the region.

In drafting this recommendation, the RTC appeared to be more concerned to stimulate recruitment of junior staff to the hospitals across the region rather than to contribute to the quality of clinical education programmes of the schools. However, it had failed to appreciate that selection of a particular location for inclusion in an existing clinical education programme was dependent on the consideration of many factors, most of which must already be in place at the location prior to an invitation to participate being made. If a potential placement met standard criteria in relation to existing staffing levels, quality of experience offered, the possibility for student supervision and assessment by suitably qualified and experienced staff, it could be considered. The writers of the report recognised that high-quality clinical education experiences are a stimulus to the recruitment of junior staff who are encouraged to seek employment in hospitals where they had gained these experiences. However, the reverse is also true – poor experiences during the clinical education programme are a strong disincentive to subsequent recruitment to the areas where these experiences were endured.

Having criticised the 'split site' arrangements made by Coventry and the ONSSP to accommodate their courses, the most important recommendation contained in the report was totally incomprehensible from an educational or a management point of view. It proposed the establishment of a 'West Midlands College of Physiotherapy' as a consortium arrangement between the three remaining schools.[14] Under the overall control of a director of physiotherapy education supported by three principals, the proposed establishment would operate on three sites with staff and students moving between them to capitalise on the strengths of each 'school'. It was further proposed that the college should operate a single course allowing for variation of the programme within the college, enabling staff and students to retain a sense of identity as well as a uniformly high standard of education. At a stroke, the PEG recommended elimination of the individual courses already developed by the schools in response to the CSP directive to establish internalised courses and required them to develop yet another course to commence within two years at the proposed new college. Finally, this new course was to be operated between three separate sites, a managerial and logistical nightmare.

The consultation period on the report lasted until 4 March 1988. Owing to the opportune publication date, the Christmas period had been spent collecting and collating responses from a variety of sources including students and clinical educators from all the clinical education bases at the SHA and NSHA hospital sites. Teaching staff, individual clinical educators, the Medical Advisory Committee at RJAH and the District Hospital Medical Committee at Shrewsbury also responded. The policy committee summarised the comments received, and prepared and submitted its official response to the proposals well within the consultation period. The school, North Staffordshire Health Authority, Shropshire Health Authority and several of the hospitals hosting components of the clinical education programme submitted further individual responses.

In making recommendations for such radical change, there had been neither indication of the potential cost of implementation of the proposals nor identification of the source of the funding that would be required to support the changes proposed. There had been no consideration of the manpower requirements for development of a totally new course in time to meet the CSP deadline of the 1989 entry. Once again, the RTC's proposals were rejected, and the PEG immediately developed another set of criteria and conducted further visits to each school before producing yet another report.

This definitive report was circulated to schools in October 1988. Having failed to gain support for proposals contained in previous reports, this one aimed to 'draw together the evidence accumulated by the Evaluation Group; encompass wherever possible the views and comments of Health Authorities; and, by analysis and reasoned argument, propose a clear, coherent Physiotherapy Training strategy for the West Midlands Region'.[15]

Each report published was larger than its predecessor had been and this one was no exception, presenting sixteen pages of text supported by seventeen appendices. Much of the information contained in the appendices was of interest, but factual inaccuracies and the bias observed in previous reports were reiterated throughout the new document.

The introduction to this latest report identified the result of the consultation period on the first report presented to the RTC by the Professional and Technical Staff Development Group in June 1986.[16] There is no record of these comments having been circulated to the schools at the time, which is unfortunate, as the schools would have been better prepared to fight recommendations contained in subsequent reports. In essence, the region remained concerned that it was contributing more than its fair share to the national pre-registration education of physiotherapists as it supported five schools of physiotherapy. This was more than any other region – most hosted one, some had two, one hosted three and several supported no school at all. It was proposed that in the future, the region should fund a training capacity that would satisfy its needs alone and, because of this, a smaller number of schools would be required. The obvious school to be targeted for closure was the ONSSP, as it was geographically the most distant from the hub of the region's activity in the Birmingham and Black Country conurbation placed relatively centrally in the region.

Fortunately, the school was not cognisant of the region's intention to close schools before the publication of the earlier reports as this would have reduced the spontaneity and vigour of the campaign to challenge and overturn the recommendations. At that time, all staff were conditioned to accept regional directives without question and not protest against perceived inequality of treatment or unfairness of judgement.

It was recommended that pre- and post-registration physiotherapy education be embraced within the framework of the Regionally Coordinated Training Services under the umbrella of the RTC.[17] This was to facilitate long-term planning with coordination of training in relation to service needs.[18] A Regional Physiotherapy Training Committee (RPTC) accountable to the RTC through the Professional and Technical Staff Development Group was to be established and schools would operate through this mechanism as soon as it was set up.

The numbers of students required annually was reviewed and in this report it was determined a suitable intake would be 160, an increase of forty from the previous report. This was to be achieved by doubling the intake at the Queen Elizabeth school and increasing to forty the intakes of Wolverhampton and Coventry schools.[19] Subject to CPSM/CSP approval being granted for these increases in student numbers, the RPTC would advise on the retention or otherwise of the Royal Orthopaedic Hospital school (ROH) and the ONSSP.[20]

The authors of the report commented favourably on the exceptionally high standard of training and education of the ROH school but indicated that some enhancement of the standard of facilities, organisation and management of the ONSSP was required. It was suggested that this be addressed and action taken as quickly as possible.[21] This followed an unofficial visit to the school by the RTO, although the UGM appeared fully conversant with the arrangements. Mr Beardwell subsequently expressed the policy committee's concerns in writing about the visit, requesting that in future both Health Authorities and the school should be advised formally of the RTO's intentions prior to his arrival at either of the school bases.[22]

A wide range of issues had been judged on this unofficial visit including: the general level of the school's facilities; the quality of furniture and fittings; the standard of orderliness and décor, and state of repair of buildings and fabric; the range and standard of equipment; the overall quality of teaching facilities available; and the general climate of the school. Almost without exception visitors to the ONSSP found it did not compare favourably with the other four schools in the region. The WMRHA RTO recommended that urgent action to remedy the perceived deficiencies should be taken by the UGM and the principal.[23]

The UGM presented a report to the December 1988 policy committee following extensive communication with the RTO and confirmed that the comments related to the Oswestry base of the school only. He indicated he would allocate approximately £20,000 for the urgent redecoration and refurbishment required. In order to make progress on the upgrading, a subcommittee consisting of the principal, Mrs Rose (a senior teacher) and a student was convened to advise on the best use of the allocated monies.[24] Upgrading was speedily effected with a practical classroom and office being converted into a smaller movement room, additional theory classroom and a storage area for movement apparatus. Seminar rooms were also provided replacing those lost in October 1986. Work was undertaken mainly at the weekends, so disruption was minimal and most equipment orders placed were speedily delivered. Some items such as notice boards for the corridor and blackout curtains for the two theory rooms and the AV room were slower to arrive. However, within a matter of months, the refurbishment and redecoration had been completed and the carpeting of the corridors, offices, library, theory classrooms and stairs immediately improved the visual impact of the school as well as making the areas more user-friendly. The additional classroom and storage facilities facilitated teaching and improved the appearance of the movement classroom, the area that had given rise to many adverse comments in the past. A plaque to commemorate the refurbishment was unveiled by Sheila Philbrook, the chairman of the CSP Council, on 30 June 1989. At the same time, following the tradition of naming rooms after people who had made a substantial contribution to the hospital, the new theory classroom was named the Mary Powell Room. This was a fitting honour to be bestowed on the last matron of the hospital, who was also a qualified physiotherapist.

Following publication of an earlier report, the WMRHA had initiated support for teacher training in the paramedical disciplines by funding four training places annually for the Cert. in Ed. component of the course. Investigation prior to the publication of this report recognised the additional pressures on schools produced by the development and implementation of courses with internalisation of assessment procedures and recommended funding three training places annually for physiotherapy to facilitate additional teacher recruitment.[25]

The RTC received all comments and submissions in relation to the report and made its final judgement on 20 February 1989. The DHSS had requested schools to increase their intakes without incurring additional expenditure[26] and the significant capital investment required to double the intake to the Queen Elizabeth school obviously influenced the final decision. The RTC determined that it would:

- establish a Regional Physiotherapy Training and Education Committee (RPTEC) as soon as practicable
- retain all schools and attempt to increase student intakes to the level requested by the DHSS without major capital investment
- establish physiotherapy education and training as a regionally coordinated service
- continue current arrangements for the training of physiotherapy teachers.

The most significant change was the establishment of the Regional Physiotherapy Training Council (RPTC), which was to perform a strategic, monitoring and resource enabling role in physiotherapy education. Both pre- and post-registration education would be embraced within the framework of regionally coordinated training services under the umbrella of the Regional Training Council. The RPTC would be accountable to the RTC through the Professional and Technical Staff Development Group to facilitate long term planning and coordination of physiotherapy training in relation to service needs and priorities.[27]

NOTES

[1] *Physiotherapy Manpower Needs – West Midlands Region*, Staff Development Group Report, June 1986

[2] WMRTC Staff Development Group (Professional and Technical Staffs) Physiotherapy Evaluation Group Interim Statement – *Outcome of Visits to Schools of Physiotherapy in the West Midlands Region*, June 1987

[3] Ibid

[4] *Physiotherapy Manpower Needs,* June 1986, op. cit.

[5] Extract from letter dated 29 June 1987 from Mr Spencer, Chairman of the Evaluation Group, to Mrs Tidswell

[6] Extracts from the minutes of the emergency ONSSP Policy Committee meeting, 27 July 1987

[7] Ibid

[8] Staff Development Group (Professional and Technical Staffs) Physiotherapy Evaluation Group Report, December 1987

[9] Reference to discussions between the CSP and government concerning the possible inclusion of physiotherapy in the Education Bill being drafted

[10] Item 7.1 of the Staff Development Group (Professional and Technical Staffs) Physiotherapy Evaluation Group Report, December 1987

[11] Item 5.2.1 of the Staff Development Group (Professional and Technical Staffs) Physiotherapy Evaluation Group Report, December 1987

[12] Item 7.8 of the Staff Development Group (Professional and Technical Staffs) Physiotherapy Evaluation Group Report, December 1987

[13] Item 7.1.2 of the Staff Development Group (Professional and Technical Staffs) Physiotherapy Evaluation Group Report, December 1987

[14] Item 5.2.3 of the Staff Development Group (Professional and Technical Staffs) Physiotherapy Evaluation Group Report, December 1987

[15] West Midlands Regional Training Services (Training and Education Section) – *Report on Physiotherapy Training in the West Midlands Region*, August 1988

[16] *Physiotherapy Manpower Needs*, June 1986, op. cit.

[17] Item 8.2 of the WMRTS (Training and Education Section) Report on Physiotherapy Training in the West Midlands Region, August 1988

[18] Item 8.3 of the WMRTS (Training and Education Section) Report on Physiotherapy Training in the West Midlands Region, August 1988

[19] Item 8.4 and 8.5 of the WMRTS (Training and Education Section)

Report on Physiotherapy Training in the West Midlands Region, August 1988

[20] Item 8.6 of the WMRTS (Training and Education Section) Report on Physiotherapy Training in the West Midlands Region, August 1988

[21] Items 8.6 and 7.14.5 of the WMRTS (Training and Education Section) Report on Physiotherapy Training in the West Midlands Region, August 1988

[22] Extracts from the minutes of the ONSSP Policy Committee meeting, 7 July 1988

[23] Letter from the WMRHA RTO to the principal of ONSSP, 2 November 1988.

[24] Extracts from the minutes of the ONSSP Policy Committee meeting, 1 December 1988

[25] Item 7.6 of the WMRTS (Training and Education Section) Report on Physiotherapy Training in the West Midlands Region, August 1988

[26] Letter from the NHS Executive concerning physiotherapy training, 17 February 1989

[27] Item 8.2 and 8.3 of West Midlands Regional Training Services, Report on Physiotherapy Training in the West Midlands Region, August 1988

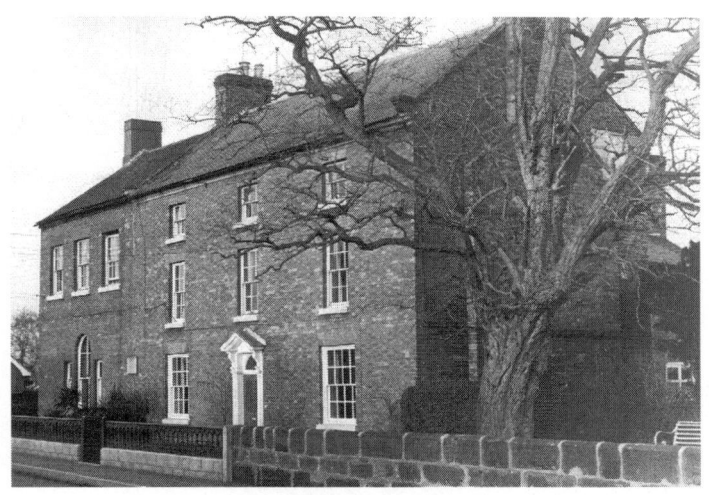

Florence House, Baschurch, the base for the Baschurch Convalescent Home between 1900 and 1921.
Reproduced by courtesy of the Shropshire Star.

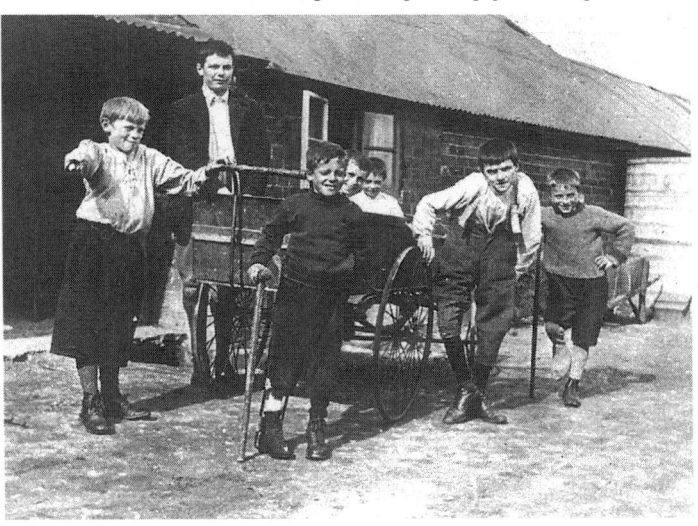

Some of the first patients of the Baschurch Convalescent Home.
Reproduced by courtesy of the Shropshire Star.

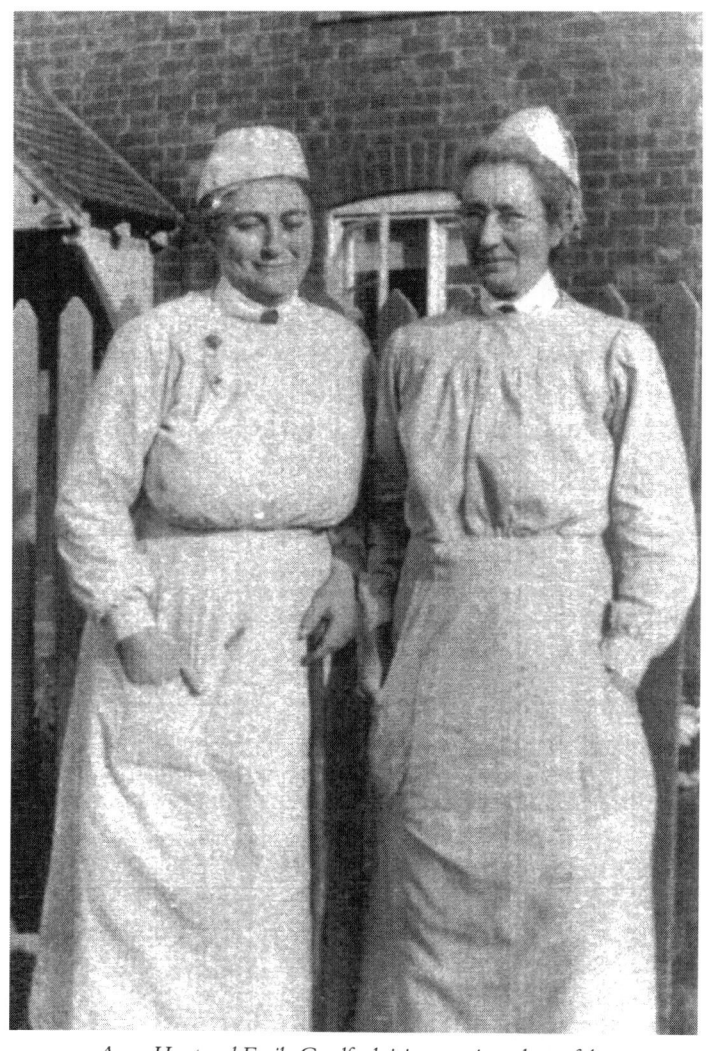

*Agnes Hunt and Emily Goodford, joint superintendents of the
Baschurch Convalescent Home.
Reproduced by courtesy of the Robert Jones and Agnes Hunt
Orthopaedic and District NHS Trust.*

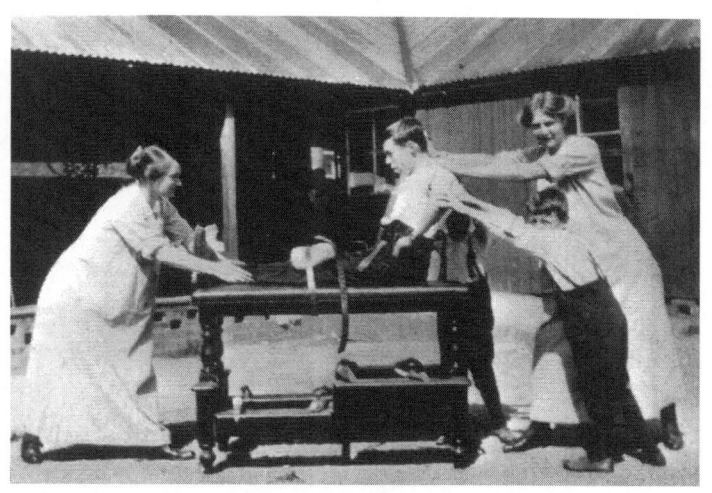

A patient assists massage staff to treat a young person with lower limb problems.
Reproduced by courtesy of the Robert Jones and Agnes Hunt
Orthopaedic and District NHS Trust.

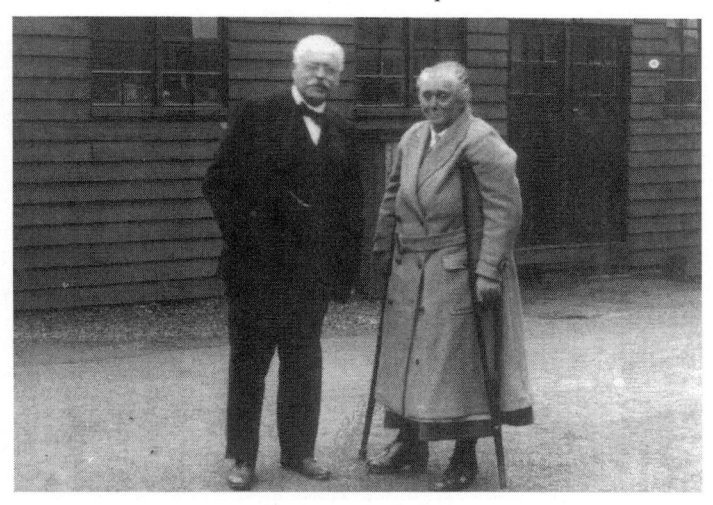

Dame Agnes Hunt and Sir Robert Jones at the Shropshire Orthopaedic Hospital, 1927.
Reproduced by courtesy of the Robert Jones and Agnes Hunt
Orthopaedic and District NHS Trust.

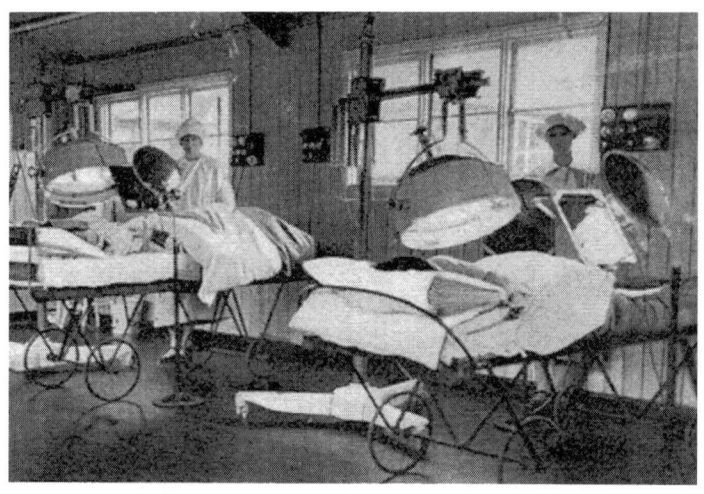

*Light treatment of patients at the Shropshire Orthopaedic Hospital, 1922.
Reproduced by courtesy of the Robert Jones and Agnes Hunt
Orthopaedic and District NHS Trust.*

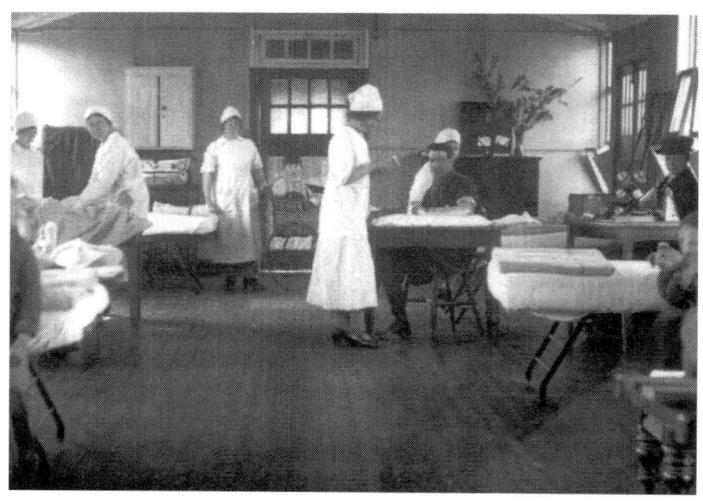

*Physiotherapy department at the Shropshire Orthopaedic Hospital, 1922.
Reproduced by courtesy of the Robert Jones and Agnes Hunt
Orthopaedic and District NHS Trust.*

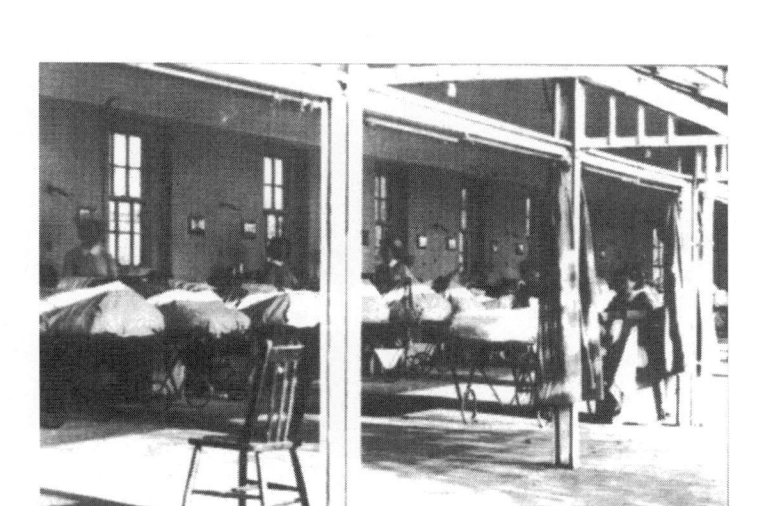

*An open-sided ward at the Shropshire Orthopaedic Hospital.
Reproduced by courtesy of the Robert Jones and Agnes Hunt
Orthopaedic and District NHS Trust.*

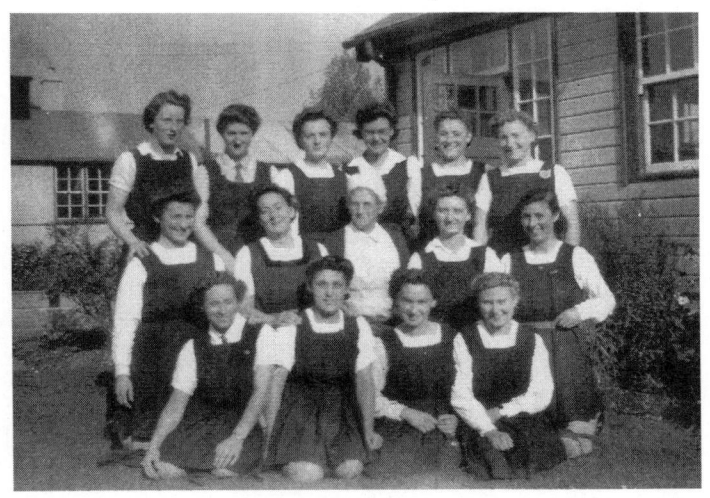

*Physiotherapy students with Miss Dalton, their principal (middle of the second row), 1939.
Reproduced by courtesy of the Robert Jones and Agnes Hunt
Orthopaedic and District NHS Trust.*

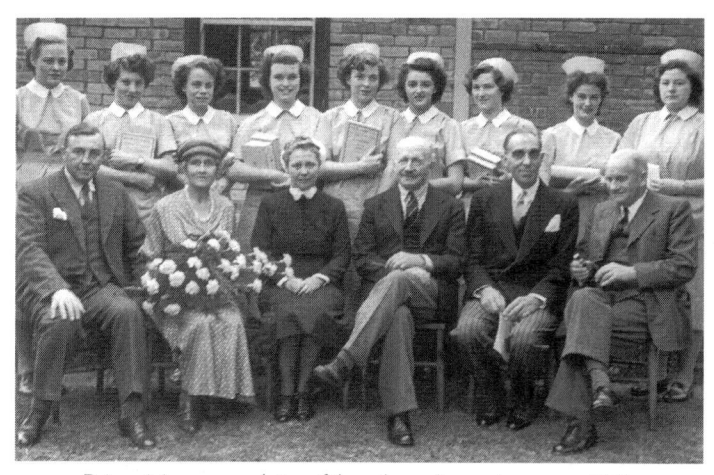

Prize-giving on completion of the orthopaedic nursing course, 1949. These students qualified as physiotherapists in 1952. Reproduced by courtesy of the Robert Jones and Agnes Hunt Orthopaedic and District NHS Trust.

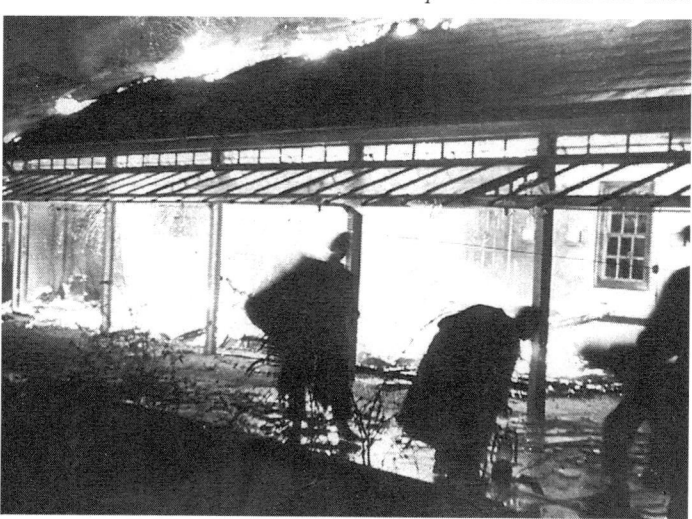

The hospital fire, January 1948. Reproduced by courtesy of the Oswestry and Border Counties Advertiser.

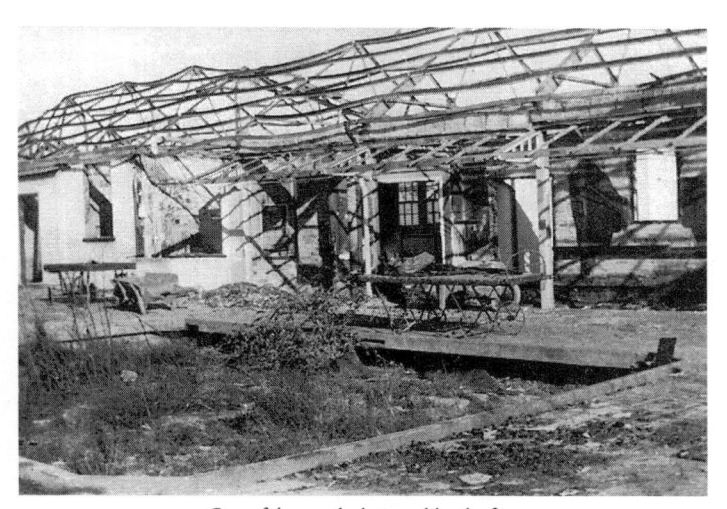

One of the wards destroyed by the fire.
Reproduced by courtesy of the Oswestry and Border Counties Advertiser.

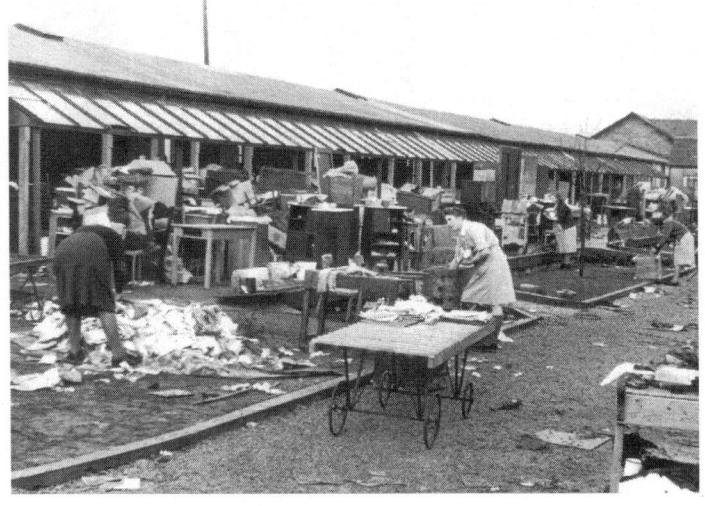

Clearing up after the fire.
Reproduced by courtesy of the Robert Jones and Agnes Hunt
Orthopaedic and District NHS Trust.

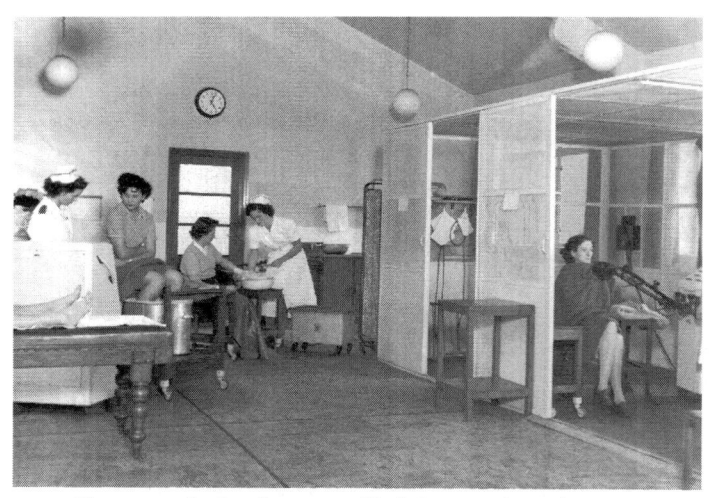

Treatments using low frequency and high frequency electrical currents.
Reproduced by courtesy of the Robert Jones and Agnes Hunt
Orthopaedic and District NHS Trust.

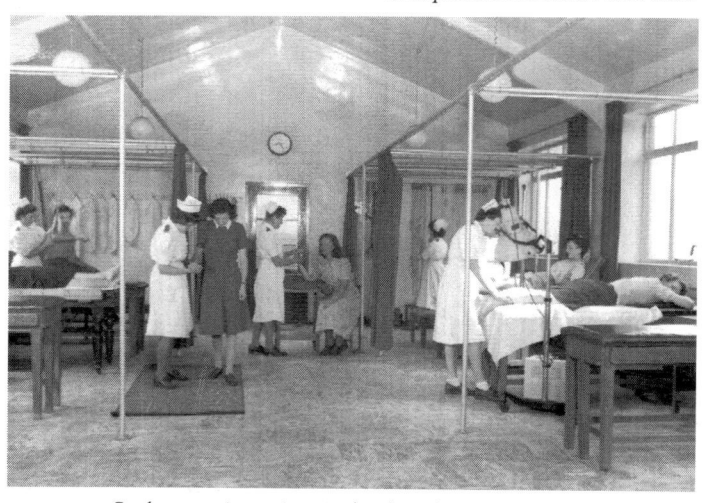

Students treating patients in the physiotherapy department.
Reproduced by courtesy of the Robert Jones and Agnes Hunt
Orthopaedic and District NHS Trust.

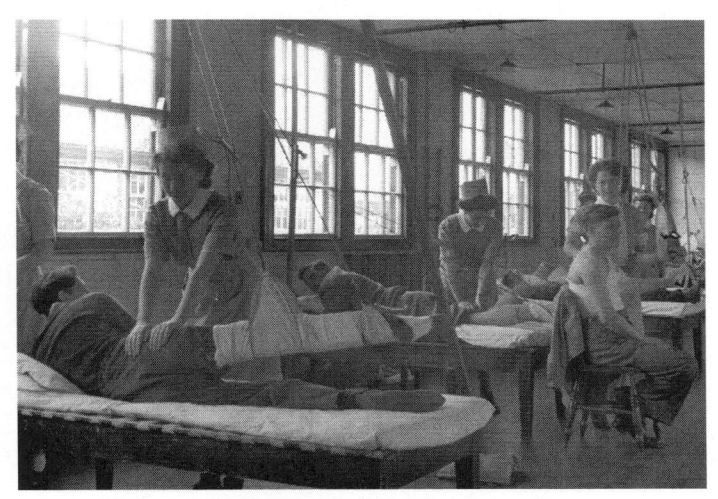

Sling suspension assists exercise in the physiotherapy department.
Reproduced by courtesy of the Robert Jones and Agnes Hunt
Orthopaedic and District NHS Trust.

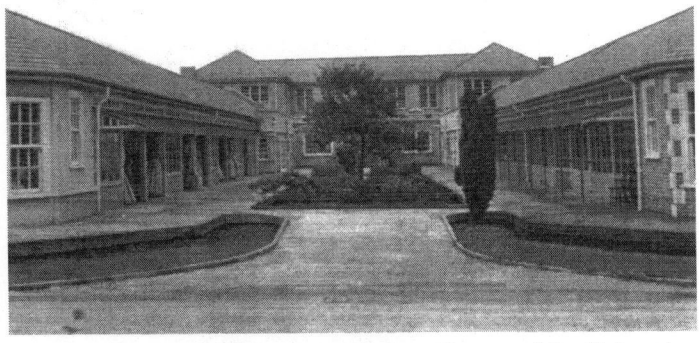

The new School of Physiotherapy viewed between Kenyon and Goodford wards,
rebuilt after the fire.
Reproduced by courtesy of the Robert Jones and Agnes Hunt
Orthopaedic and District NHS Trust.

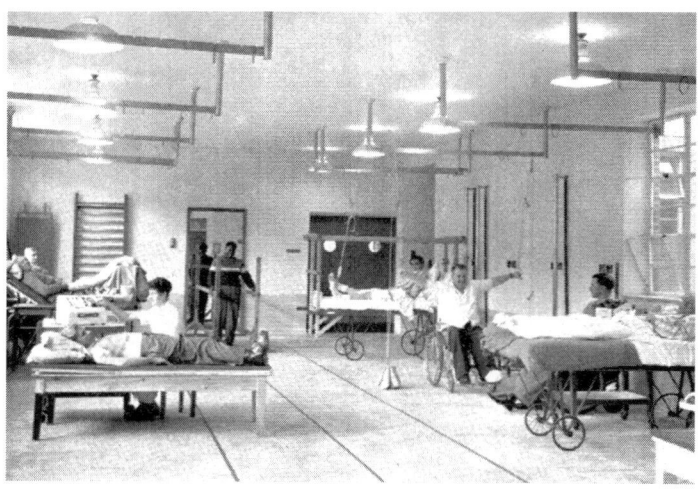

*Treatments in the new physiotherapy department.
Reproduced by courtesy of the Robert Jones and Agnes Hunt
Orthopaedic and District NHS Trust.*

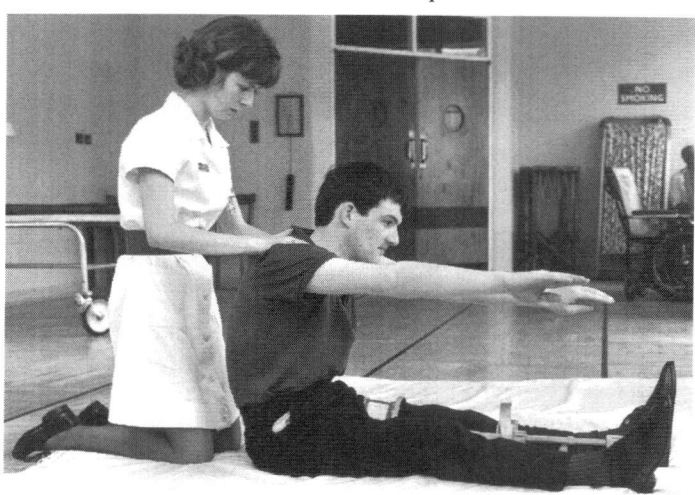

*Re-education of balance in the physiotherapy department, 1970s.
Reproduced by courtesy of the Robert Jones and Agnes Hunt
Orthopaedic and District NHS Trust.*

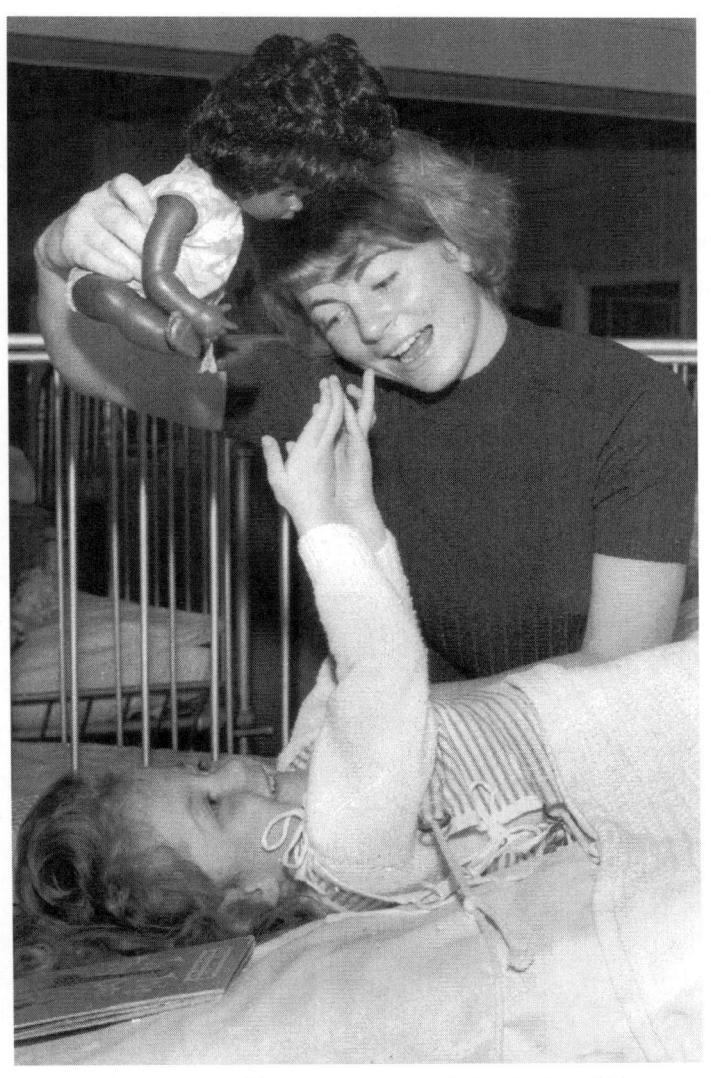

*A physiotherapy student exercises a young patient on traction, 1970s.
Reproduced by courtesy of the Robert Jones and Agnes Hunt
Orthopaedic and District NHS Trust.*

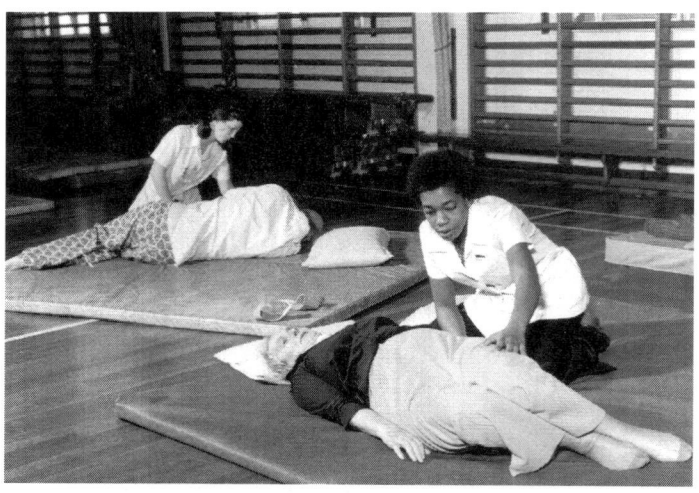

Mat exercises in the gymnasium, 1970s.
Reproduced by courtesy of the Robert Jones and Agnes Hunt
Orthopaedic and District NHS Trust.

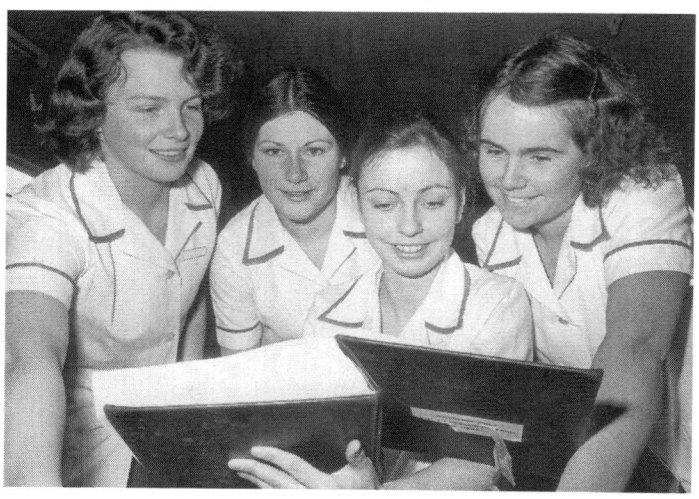

Students raised a substantial sum of money for the Spinal Injuries Unit by a sponsored read of Gray's Anatomy, 1977.
Reproduced by courtesy of the Shropshire Star.

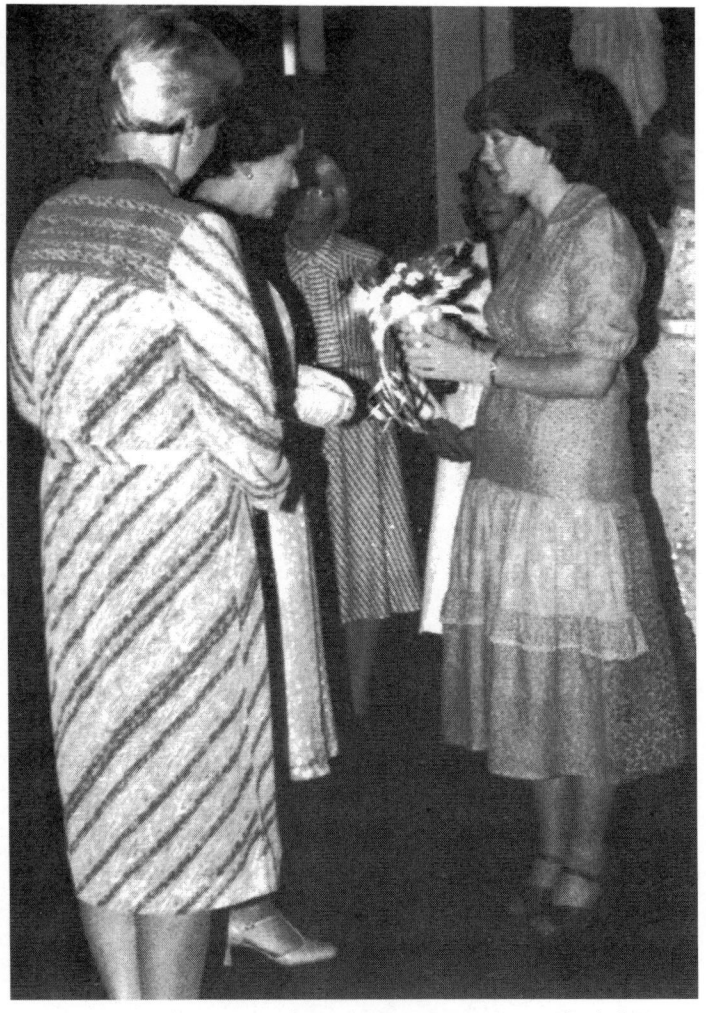

A second year student presents a bouquet to Her Majesty Queen Elizabeth II at a reception to celebrate the diamond jubilee of the award of the Royal Charter to the Chartered Society of Physiotherapy, 1980.
Reproduced by courtesy of the Robert Jones and Agnes Hunt Orthopaedic and District NHS Trust.

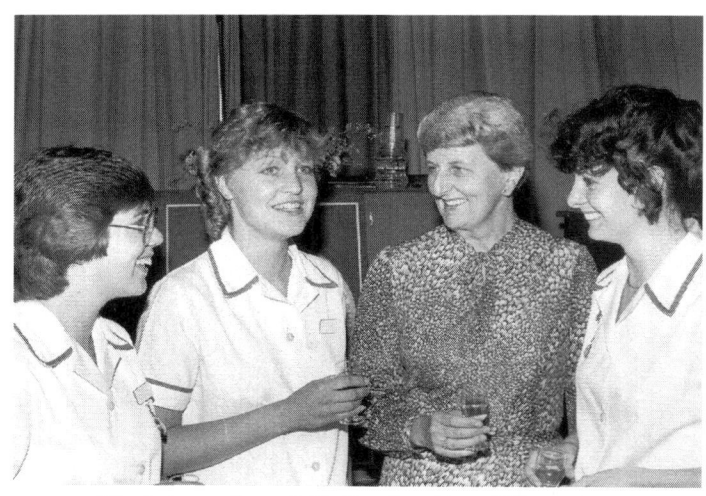

The chairman of council, Ida Bromley with qualifying students at the badge-giving ceremony in June 1982.
Reproduced by courtesy of the Shropshire Star.

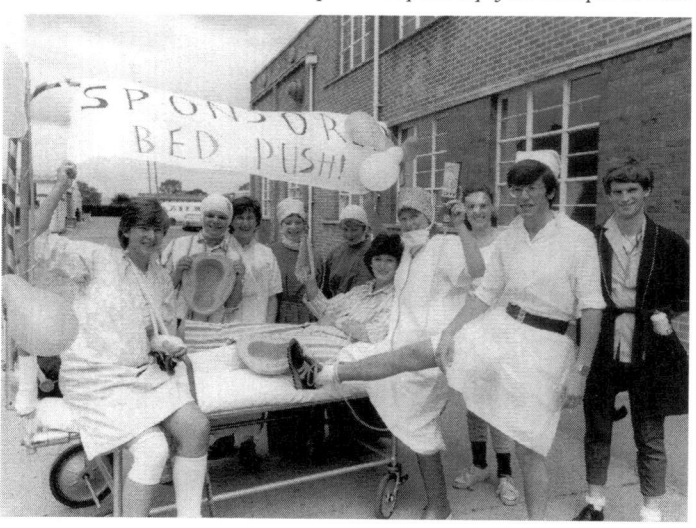

Fund-raising bed push by student physiotherapists in 1984.
Reproduced by courtesy of the Oswestry and Border Counties Advertiser.

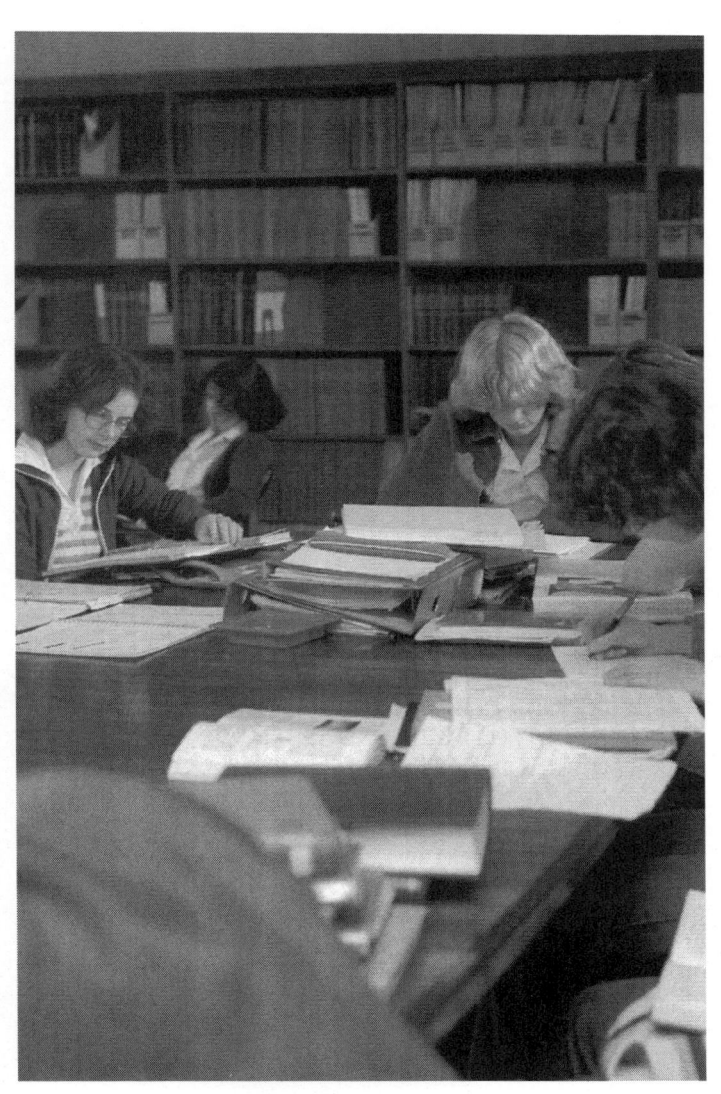

*Study in the Institute Library.
Reproduced by courtesy of the Robert Jones and Agnes Hunt
Orthopaedic and District NHS Trust.*

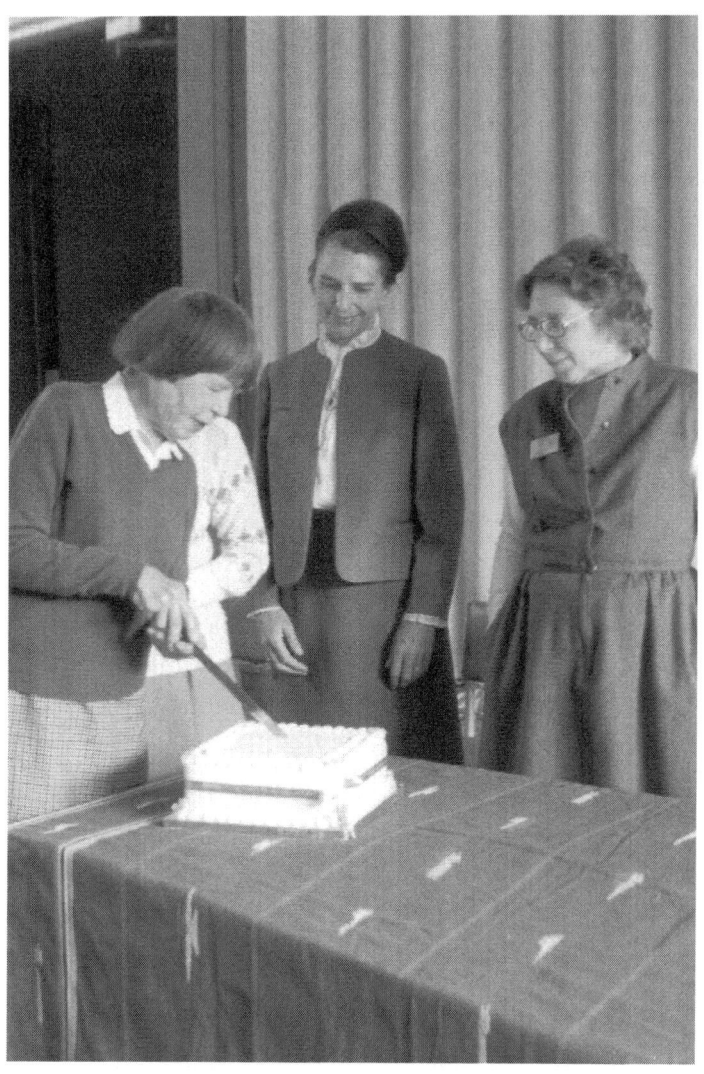

Miss Anderson cuts the cake to celebrate the fortieth anniversary of the establishment of the Old Oswestrian Physiotherapists' Association, watched by Wyn Cannell and Marian Tidswell, 1984.

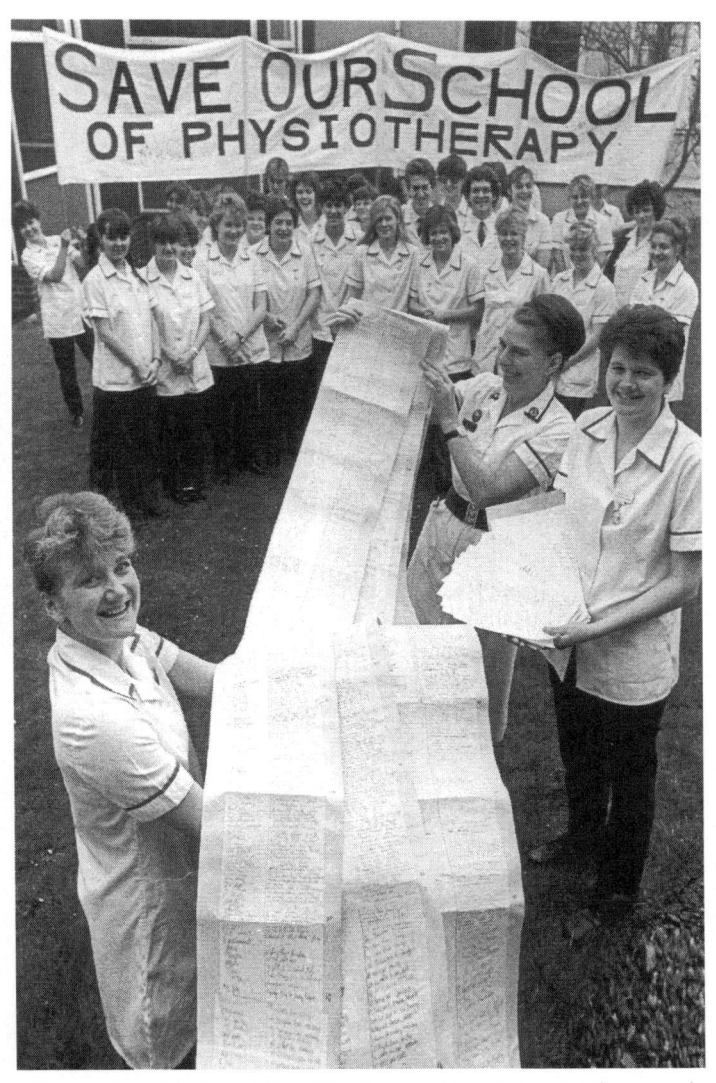

Students show the principal the petition they raised to protest against the proposed closure of the school by the Regional Health Authority, 1987.
Reproduced by courtesy of the Shropshire Star.

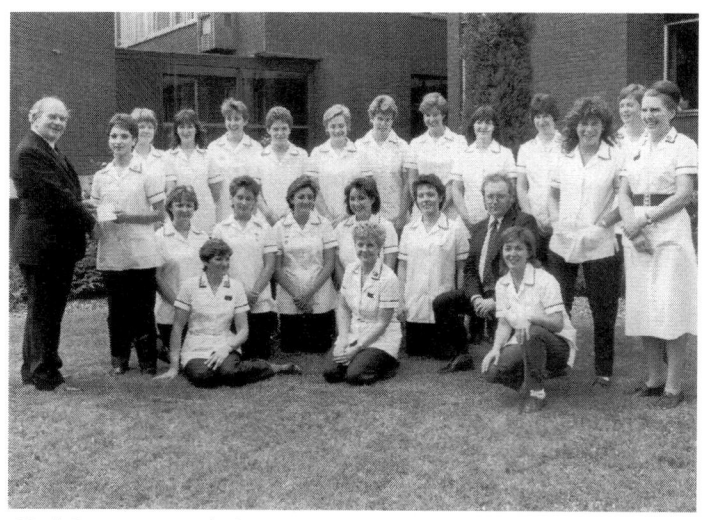

Hugh Davies presents the first Jean Davies Memorial prize to Lucy Oliver, 1985.
Reproduced by courtesy of the Oswestry and Border Counties Advertiser.

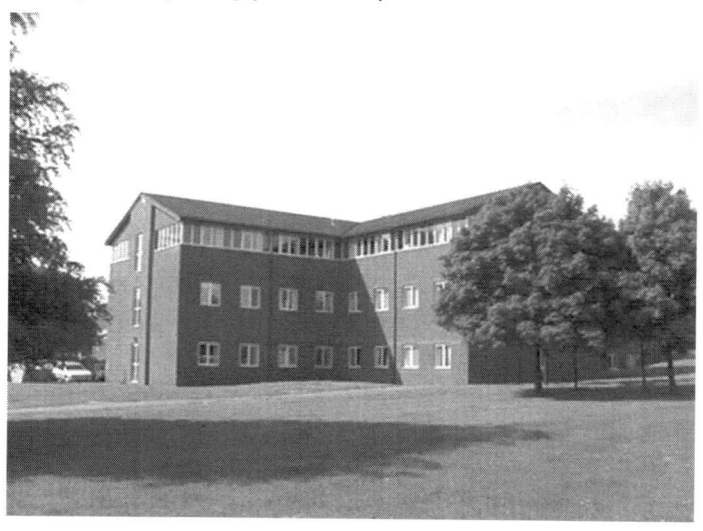

MacKay Building
Reproduced by courtesy of Keele University

Chapter 15
Course Internalisation: 1988 Onwards

The 1986–7 school year had started with the termination of proposals to mount an honours degree in physiotherapy and movement science with SPEAR and the opening of negotiations with Keele University for an honours degree in physiotherapy and management science. Being a hospital-based school, the university required a significant proportion of course teaching to be provided by campus-based departments and, as the university could not provide support in the range of subject teaching directly related to physiotherapy, it had been necessary to seek alternative relevant subject matter. Determination of an appropriate syllabus in management science was progressing well and the school was confident it could produce the completed course documentation and achieve validation prior to the CSP withdrawal of the national examinations. Planning was, however, suspended by the university on publication of the PEG's interim statement in June 1987 and the school was then left with insufficient time to complete negotiations.[1]

Over the 1986 Christmas period the additional committee structures required to support course internalisation were introduced by the establishment of ad hoc steering committees for clinical education in both Health Authorities and a course planning and review committee. The new committees included representation from teaching staff, students and clinical physiotherapists and satisfied totally the CSP's requirements. They would include university staff if and when a degree course was validated. The education committee was renamed the policy committee and granted the power to make appropriate policy decisions in relation to the school. Secretarial support of the committee, previously undertaken by Jeff Silk, now devolved to the school as the UGM considered he had neither the staff nor the resources to continue providing the required level of support.[2] Mr Beardwell, the principal's line manager, assumed managerial responsibility for the committee and the school provided administrative and secretarial support.[3] It was gratifying subsequently to receive positive feedback from NSHA about the improvement in the administration of the committee following this realignment of responsibilities.[4]

Progress had been made slowly and steadily on the proposal to produce a unified budget for the school in response to the CPSM/CSP directive. It had been fraught with difficulties as it involved the apportionment of monies by each of the two funding Health Authorities arguably to support activities that were to be undertaken outwith their individual boundaries. Agreement was eventually reached mid 1987 at the time when SHA was decentralising district-based clinical budgets and returning the responsibility for these services to the units.[5] Naturally any attempt to decentralise the school budget in SHA would jeopardise its viability as it contravened CPSM directives and was opposed by the principal and the NSHA representatives on the policy committee. Reassurance was given by the SHA representatives that there was to be no decentralisation of the school's budget, nor alteration of the principal's line management, although subsequent events belied this statement. This reassertion of the school's position was against the principles of unit management and the UGM continued his attempts to gain financial and administrative control of the school.

Following the publication of the interim statement, the UGM had many unofficial meetings with teaching staff, the principal's PA and students. They invariably occurred when the principal was away from the Oswestry school base and were reported by students who had been disconcerted by the approaches and had requested the principal's presence at any future meetings. This was denied by the UGM and, after several heated exchanges between him and the principal, matters came to a head on 25 November, when he suspended the principal for two weeks pending investigation into her alleged financial mismanagement of the school's affairs. The principal's Industrial Relations representative immediately confirmed that in line with SHA standing financial instructions, the line manager was the only person with the authority to suspend an individual and, also, the alleged misdemeanours did not justify suspension. He confirmed that the UGM was not the principal's line manager; however, SHA did not reverse the action taken. At the subsequent hearing following a full investigation, the unsubstantiated allegations were withdrawn and the UGM was instructed to inform all departments within the hospital of this fact, but he failed to comply. Nine months later he sent an internal memo informing only three departments.

There were several staff changes during 1987, some scheduled and others resulting from overturn of the interim statement. These in summary are that Jean Richards became a permanent member of the teaching staff and Nora Richards returned in a part-time capacity. Shân Aguilar returned to the school on successful completion of the Cert. in Ed. course at Dudley College of Further Education to complete the Dip TP component of the course and Jane Holmes started the Dudley course as a member of the ONSSP staff. Jean Rogers returned to clinical duties and Ann Neill left the area to take up a post at the Withington school. Despite the damaging effects of the interim statement, teaching staff levels within the school had not reduced significantly and there was no uncertainty about the commitment of the staff to the next student intake.

The most significant staff change that occurred was Judy Bebb's transfer from the school to the Institute of Orthopaedics. Judy applied for a post in the institute in July when the school's future was very uncertain, although she did not take up her new position until after the embargo on the 1987 intake had been lifted. Her departure was a devastating blow to the school, but security of her future employment was of prime consideration. Leanne Woods replaced her once the recommendations of the interim statement had been overturned.[6]

Examination results are the yardstick by which the effectiveness of a course tends to be judged and, for some years, the school had been satisfied with progress in this area as each set of results published demonstrated an improvement on the previous year's performance. Concern was expressed in the staff room that 1987 would prove to be the exception owing to the stress students had experienced at the quinquennial inspection the previous October and the PEG's visit in April. However, they had appeared to take these events in their stride and, despite making frequent complaints about the loss of the seminar rooms and the inadequacy of their study facilities in the staff residency, seemed to be coping. The examination schedule was completed by the second week in June prior to publication of the interim statement and the results were awaited with some trepidation.

When published, the results in the Part 1 and Part 2 examinations were twenty-five per cent and fifteen per cent above the national average respectively. In the qualifying examination the results were particularly gratifying as a 100 per cent success rate in the patient assessment component of the examination was achieved. As one candidate only had failed to achieve a pass in Paper 1 and another in Paper 2, the performance of the cohort was exceptional. The school had produced the best results in the country and, with the success of the two retake candidates at the second diet of the examinations, all were able to attend the awards ceremony as qualified chartered physiotherapists. It was a splendid result for the students and staff and the timing was immaculate. These qualifying students were the first to gain the Graduate Diploma in Physiotherapy following the CSP's decision to separate qualification and membership, and the cohort, with great generosity and foresight, bought the school a set of the academic regalia that supported this change in the status of their qualification. Helen Atkinson, principal of the Coventry School of Physiotherapy, presented the awards at a lighthearted, enjoyable ceremony held in September.[7]

Staff who had been quite united as to the future direction to be taken by the school were, following the publication of the interim statement, somewhat divided. They determined they wished to produce a document for submission through the CSP/CPSM validation system with proposals for an internalised course. This followed the curtailment of the degree negotiations in June and was to refute the PEG's contention that the ONSSP had made no progress with course development. The policy committee was informed that the required documentation could be produced within a matter of months, but the course could not readily be implemented without an increase in the teaching establishment.[8] Mr Bloor, the principal's line manager from NSHA, objected to the proposal, identifying that if the school decided to progress with development of an internalised course instead of the degree, this would have to be reported to and agreed by the NSHA, as it would be a major policy change. NSHA would require supportive documentation giving sound reasons for internalisation.[9] It was therefore determined that the degree negotiations should continue alongside the proposals for internalisation until such time as a final decision had to be made.

Internalisation could be viewed as a very positive development as it enabled schools to be more flexible and innovative in the design of their programmes within the framework of the CSP curriculum of study. The first of these courses were presented by schools with numbers of staff sufficient to readily separate the functions of teaching, assessment, examination, marking and moderation of the different course components and resembled closely the courses they replaced.

This was not an option for the ONSSP owing to its low teaching establishment but staff determined to use internalisation to develop a viable course capitalising fully on the school's strengths. The school had been founded to provide expert physical rehabilitation to patients following months or even years of enforced bed rest by the application of the highest level of clinical expertise to optimise patient recovery and independence in the most efficient manner. The development of a high level of clinical competence and confidence remained at the core of the existing ONSSP course with academic components supporting, strengthening and consolidating the development of clinical excellence. Despite the traditionally low teaching establishment, each member of the tutorial staff had, until 1974, been in charge of a defined ward or clinical area in either Shropshire or North Staffordshire. Clinical involvement was reduced somewhat following implementation of the Halsbury Report,[10] when roles and responsibilities of all physiotherapists were redefined. School staff had maintained clinical contact by liaison with clinicians, treatment of selected patients and supervision of students in areas of their clinical specialism and/or preferences. The CPSM/CSP inspectors at their visits in 1983 and 1986[11] applauded this level of commitment although they advised staff to be vigilant to ensure clinical responsibilities did not interfere with necessary course development.

Clinical staff at both sites had strong connections with the school and since 1980 had worked unceasingly to restructure and improve the means by which clinical competence was developed during the course. By 1987, a comprehensive progressive clinical education programme was in place that clinical staff had developed in partnership with the school. Clinical educators were confident and competent in all aspects of student supervision and clinical teaching, and were experts in course and student clinical assessment, evaluation and review.

Ken Stopani, Philip Holbourn and Marian Tidswell presented the first of the school's proposals for internalisation to the Joint Validation and Recognition Panel (V&R panel) on 5 November and although panel members commented favourably on the philosophy underlying the presentation, the course was not accepted.[12] Unfortunately, in their haste to present the course, staff had not followed the CSP-published procedure for submission of documentation, essential with such an innovative model. Initially an outline of the proposed course should be submitted and, on its approval by the V&R panel, submission of the complete documentation would be requested. The letter from CSP dated 23 November 1987 reminded staff of this procedure.[13]

Relatively undaunted by this initial rejection, staff took heed of the CSP's comments, accepted their advice and submitted an outline of the proposed course to the panel for consideration at their meeting on 10 February 1988.[14] Ken Stopani and Cath Rose presented the outline and were distressed to learn that it was still not considered acceptable. The panel suggested the school develop alternative ideas for the course before resubmission of any further documentation. Unfortunately, no written confirmation of these comments survives and, when the outcome of the resubmission was reported to the policy committee, Mr Bloor and Mr Beardwell, the principal's line managers, offered to participate in future negotiations over the course to ensure complete understanding of requirements by all parties.[15] This suggestion was accepted gratefully, not least by the principal, who was recovering from injuries received in a road traffic accident and was not likely to return to duty for several months.

Over the next weeks, significant correspondence was exchanged and staff endeavoured to modify their proposals, not only to satisfy CSP requirements, but also to ensure the additional stresses imposed by the course could be accommodated from within the school's limited staff resources. Sadly, although a revised version of the course outline gained acceptance by the CSP in May 1988,[16] much of the innovation and imagination of the initial proposal was lost. Staff were invited to submit the complete documentation to the November V&R panel, incorporating all the suggestions that had been made for clarification and expansion of several areas of the outline to explain how the course would be implemented.

Marian returned to duty during September and accompanied Ken Stopani, Jean Richards and Cath Rose to the V&R panel meeting. Ken, Jean and Cath had developed the course during her absence and confidently presented the proposal. After all the contact and support they had been given by CSP during the course development and their close adherence to procedural guidelines, they anticipated a positive response from the panel. This, however, was not to be as the panel requested a further rewrite of the document with less detail and with some reordering of content, but required no changes to the course structure or its assessment procedures.[17] The panel proposed the documentation should be resubmitted in May 1989.

Panel decisions were normally decisive, giving clear guidance to a school as to what was required, but the decision made on this occasion belied the process and appeared to be nothing more than a delaying tactic. Several courses had gained acceptance on the promise of subsequent modification of documentation or with minor procedural changes and the refusal to grant approval when no significant change was required could not realistically be justified. The school was, however, then facing another closure attempt following publication of a further report from the West Midlands Regional Training Council published in August 1988,[18] which makes the panel's actions more understandable.

A further set of course documentation was produced and submitted to the panel in May 1989 and this time the submission gained acceptance with course approval being granted for five years. The school received confirmation of the result from the CPSM[19] and the CSP[20] following a visit to review the available facilities. Additional clinical placements were required to allow full sequencing of the clinical education programme and these were negotiated successfully prior to the start of the course in September. When the course was finally granted approval, Eva Jahn and Nigel Palastanga, principals from the Royal Orthopaedic Hospital and the Cardiff schools respectively, were appointed and approved as external examiners.

Staff spent the summer break developing the handbooks and student guides for each year of the course and preparatory work for the examinations was undertaken. Initially individual questions were submitted by all members of staff and shredded by a senior staff member prior to construction of the papers. Staff worked in groups of three in the preparation of three question papers for each examination. When the papers were considered to be balanced, of equal difficulty and met the published objectives for the examination, they were sent to the external examiners for approval. Following acceptance of the written papers, a similar process was followed for preparation of the practical examinations.

To reduce the very real concerns about the small staff numbers concerned in the project, alternative means of funding additional teaching posts were explored. The policy committee agreed that, if overseas fee-paying students could be recruited, a portion of the fees they paid could be used to fund additional staff.[21] The proposal was welcomed although it was recognised there would be several months' time lag before recruitment of additional teaching staff could be considered, which did not ease the current situation. In the event, only one privately funded student was recruited for the 1988 cohort and, although subsequently the numbers recruited were more encouraging, there was never sufficient additional money to support an extra member of staff.

Towards the end of 1987 the school's staffing position had improved to the extent that it expected to be fully staffed on establishment by the end of the year. This situation was very welcome as staff at that time were still attempting to produce the course document for an internalised course that would satisfy the CSP. Subsequently, on implementation of the internalised course they would have to maintain the teaching and examination requirements for both courses being run by the school for two years. However, by the end of 1987, the northern unit of SHA was in financial difficulty and imposed a 2.5 per cent vacancy factor savings requirement on all departments in the hospital.[22] It appeared financial and administrative responsibility for the school had been transferred from district to unit level in SHA although there had been no consultation about, or agreement to, the change. In the absence of any written evidence of the realignment of administrative and budget responsibilities, the principal continued to operate the school as a district-managed resource and, as such, queried why it was subjected to the unit's saving's targets. No answer was forthcoming, only reiteration of the need to take action to avoid exceeding establishment post-occupancy.

Following the UGM's warning that the school would have 6.88 staff in post against an establishment of 7.11 by the end of the year, drastic action was taken to maintain the school within its current establishment. The first loss was that of a qualified teacher, Kim Jones, who had intended to join the staff in January 1988. In view of the uncertainties of her potential contract position at the ONSSP, she took a post in another school. The second loss was Shân Aguilar. On qualification as a teacher in December 1987, she had initially been offered a full-time permanent contract at the school. This was changed to a temporary renewable contract when the staff recruitment restrictions were imposed and she felt so insecure with the arrangement that she left the school in August 1988. Jane Holmes returned to the school in September 1988 to undergo the final term of her teacher training course and wished to be employed by the school on qualification. With Shân's departure in August, this was possible; also, with the gap between the two appointments, the required vacancy factor saving was achieved.

The school's application for funding to train a student teacher in 1988 was rejected and, as there was insufficient money within the school's budget to fund the post, once Jane qualified it was without a student teacher in training for the first time since 1980. This embargo lasted for one year only and the school was offered sponsorship for Jean Bourne to train as a teacher on the 1989 course.[23] Jean had extensive managerial experience and had completed a master's degree at Keele University. With this qualification she would boost yet further the academic profile of the ONSSP staff. Changes in the office personnel were also accommodated during 1988 as Karen Bright and Leanne Woods left during the spring term to be replaced by Caroline Meeks and Elaina Evans. Elaina and Caroline quickly developed a good rapport with students and staff and formed a loyal and hardworking team that carried the school through the remaining years of RTC activity in relation to the rationalisation of physiotherapy education provision in the West Midlands region.

Teaching staff continued to take advantage of the personal development made possible by retention of the school's training budget and, in September 1988, Marilyn started a master's course in education at Manchester University and Marian and Ken started a master's course in medical ethics at Keele University. The acquisition of additional qualifications by staff was necessary if the school was ultimately to be accepted into the university environment and the knowledge gained by the courses was of immediate benefit to both the school and the individuals concerned. Staff gained an improved body of knowledge and developed a more questioning approach to their work; students benefited from the improved academic orientation to physiotherapy being developed in the school.

The stress imposed by the recommendations for closure of the school had a deleterious effect on the results of the first diet of qualifying examinations in 1988. This was disappointing after the successes of the previous year, but quite understandable as this was the cohort that had borne the brunt of the initial RTC activity and had been subjected to considerable disruption by the frequent visits by members of the PEG. All were successful at retake. The 100 per cent success of the 1987 cohort in Part 1 was a just reward for the efforts made to permit the school to accept them. Students continued to support the school with fund-raising activities and in March 1989 they held a sponsored massage for Comic Relief that raised over £300.[24] As the activity provided a full day's voluntary practice of techniques taught in the classroom, the students involved benefited as much as the charity to which the funds were donated. They also held a coffee morning to boost student funds and ran a sponsored car wash, which was very popular with hospital staff.

Changes were proposed and implemented during 1989 concerning the school base at Haywood Hospital in Stoke-on-Trent. This had not been used for regular formal teaching since introduction of the block system some years previously and now was required by other departments with more pressing teaching and training needs. It was determined that the ONSSP base should be relocated in the hospital centre and would provide the school with improved accommodation on a more suitable site than Haywood Hospital.[25] When the move was completed, students were within walking distance of the majority of their clinical education placements so the need for hospital transport was reduced significantly. They also had access to the medical library, a lecture room if required and areas where they could study without distraction.

After the 100 per cent success of the 1987 cohort in the first diet of the Part 1 examinations, it was hoped the cohort taking the last of these examinations in 1989 would be equally successful. When the results were published, one candidate was found to have achieved distinction and one had failed at the first attempt, although was successful on retake. The Part 2 results that year were remarkably good considering the uncertainties of the school's position during the majority of their course. Eleven of the nineteen candidates entered for the examination qualified at the first attempt. One student had already delayed entry due to injuries received in a road traffic accident and so, in September, the examinations were completed by the eight retake students and one taking them for the first time. A further six students qualified at this time. One achieved a distinction in patient assessment, one student failed Paper 1 a second time and another Paper 2. The student entering for the first time was successful in Paper 1 but failed the other two components of the examination. These three candidates were scheduled to make another attempt to qualify in June 1990.[26]

The internalised course was implemented in autumn 1989 with an initial cohort of twenty-two. Unfortunately, course implementation coincided with further financial constraints imposed by the northern unit with a requirement to make another one per cent saving on existing budgets. As only two self-funded students had been accepted on to the course, there was no possibility of using surplus monies to fund an additional teacher and the school was required to reduce expenditure at a time when increased resources were urgently required. When staff actually started the new course, the reality of the additional workload became immediately obvious despite the preparatory work that had been undertaken over the summer months.

During the autumn term Jean Richards prepared and implemented a training course for clinical educators to replace the previous course operated by the region that had been discontinued. It consisted of a series of workshops on topics such as assessment, learning in the clinical situation, setting of treatment goals, counselling, evaluation of student performance and report writing.[27] Clinical educators attended the course during their normal working hours and the course fee was waived. This reduced significantly the costs of running the course with the small additional financial assistance required covered by the training budgets in the location where the course was being held.

Staff worked to the limit of their capabilities to implement the new teaching and assessment schedules, prepare examinations for the second year of the internalised course and maintain teaching, assessment and support of the two cohorts taking CSP examinations. Generous support was given by the two external examiners and the additional stress imposed by their presence at the school was more than outweighed by the guidance, support and encouragement given freely at each visit.

Another change that predicted an increase in the workload that had to be absorbed at this time was alteration of the student recruitment process. The CSP decided that, as many physiotherapy courses were now proceeding to degree status and used the UCCA system for recruitment, maintenance of their Central Admissions Unit was uneconomic and schools still implementing graduate diploma courses would have to subscribe to PCAS, the alternative recruitment agency for non-degree courses.[28]

Students were significantly distressed by three arson attacks that occurred in the staff residency during the year, when property was destroyed but, fortunately, no one was injured. The UGM determined that one of the physiotherapy students was the arsonist, but as she had been a ward patient at the time of the first fire, immobilised by continuous cervical traction, it was inconceivable that she could have been responsible. However, the day after the third fire, she was arrested and subjected to eight hours' gruelling interrogation at Oswestry police station. Following this, the UGM contacted the principal demanding the student's immediate expulsion from the school. The student had, of course, denied involvement in the incidents and was now to be released on police bail. She was to be excluded from the staff residency and it was proposed she be given a bed on a ward for the night to enable close supervision prior to her imminent departure from the hospital. In the event, with police approval, the student spent the night at the principal's home after her ordeal and subsequently completed her course on schedule, entering the profession of her choice on qualification. Hospitals are notorious places for rumour and several senior staff at the hospital suspected the identity of the perpetrator of the fires. Nothing was ever proven, but as no fires were set once this person left the hospital, their suspicions appeared to be confirmed. Despite these additional problems, the academic year progressed and students held another most successful conference for representatives from all the UK schools of physiotherapy in March 1990.

Students taking the Part 2 qualifying examinations this year were the 1987 intake and, following their 100 per cent success in the Part 1 examination, their qualifying examination results were also very impressive. Fourteen of the seventeen-strong cohort qualified at the first attempt, gaining two distinctions in patient assessment, one in Paper 1 and four in Paper 2. One entrant had been unsuccessful in Paper 2 and two had failed the patient assessment; however, all were successful at the second attempt. Eileen Frith, a mature student from New Zealand, was awarded the Jean Davies prize in June. Eileen, who also gained a distinction in patient assessment, was a very popular choice and, as her background, experience and timing of physiotherapy education matched that of Jean, she was a worthy recipient of the prize.[29] The cohort had more than justified their presence at the school and had been a very supportive group. Marian was a little surprised and humbled by their request that she should present the awards at their ceremony in September, but was honoured to do so.

Two students taking failed components of the Part 2 examinations for the third time were successful; however, the entrant still recovering from a major road traffic accident was advised to take several months off for recuperation before making her third and final attempt to qualify before cessation of the CSP examinations.[30]

The results of the promotional examination for the first cohort taking the internalised course were equally pleasing with the majority of the entrants achieving success; one gained distinction and one failed. The entrant who failed withdrew from the course prior to the retake examination. One member of this cohort had deferred entry to the examination owing to family illness and was successful at the second attempt at the examination.[31] Staff had been initially sceptical about the preparation of three matched sets of papers for each scheduled examination. They were now convinced this level of preparedness was essential, as circumstances had dictated that all prepared papers for this first promotional examination had been used.

All that remained to complete the first year was for the external examiners to write their report for submission to the CSP and for the school to prepare its evaluation report to complete the first course report of the internalised course. The end of year reports by the external examiners, also included in the course report, recognised that staff industry and enthusiasm had resulted in effective implementation of the course with few teething troubles. Some adjustments to timetabling, sequencing of teaching and the

OSPE examination stations were discussed and implemented for the following cohort.[32] Students commented that distribution of the workload had been patchy and made suggestions and requests for improved timetabling. It was considered that the overall balance of the course was good with some overlap between movement and biomechanics. Cath Rose prepared the first course report prior to leaving to take a post at the Liverpool school. Her resignation was a disappointing decision as she had been a prime mover in the development and implementation of the course and it had been hoped she would follow at least one cohort to qualification. However, her departure made it possible to employ Jean Bourne once she qualified as a teacher in December. Barbara Hollins, a musculoskeletal expert, started the Cert. in Ed. course in September 1990 with regional sponsorship.

Owing to unexpected losses due to health problems during the first weeks of the course, the second cohort was reduced to twenty-one from the twenty-three who started. Staff and student satisfaction was much higher for this group than the first cohort as all the comments and criticisms raised in the first course report by students, staff and the external examiners had been acted on. Performance in the promotional examination at the end of the year also improved on the first cohort's achievement as eighteen candidates were successful at the first attempt, three gaining distinction. The remaining three candidates succeeded at the second attempt.[33]

External examiners visited students on clinical secondment during the second year in addition to monitoring the assessment process. Several placements were visited and the examiners commented on the high level of commitment of both the academic staff and clinical educators whose approach was orientated to meeting student needs. Clinical educators were welcoming and positive throughout the visits and students were interested and committed to the course. By the end of the year, seventeen candidates had achieved a pass mark in course work, three of them with distinction. Two candidates were of fail grade at this stage; one of them completed the course successfully, the other repeated the second year before discontinuing her studies.

The external examiners commented that the course had

developed well over the year due to the determination of the staff to make it succeed and their sheer hard work. The marking schemes for assessments were clearly defined and the marks allocated to students were considered to be fair. The atmosphere surrounding the course was now much more relaxed and a genuine feeling of cooperation existed between the external examiners and the course team. The principal and staff were congratulated on the high standard being maintained in the course.[34]

The academic year 1991–2 saw the completion of the initial run of the graduate diploma with internalised assessment procedures. As in previous years, the external examiners were very supportive, visiting the school for observation of clinical education assessments and the final clinical examination; they also moderated the different forms of written assessment presented as coursework, assignment or examination. This was the first year for students to qualify and it is rewarding to note that all the candidates who entered the final examination were successful albeit that two required a second attempt to satisfy the examiners in the clinical examination. Several distinctions were awarded across the range of assessment procedures. The course had been planned to allow students with different abilities to demonstrate their knowledge by using a range of assessment methods rather than by adhering to the previously established standard examination formats. The results proved that this was a successful approach as individual students appeared to excel in the assessment format suited to their particular requirements. The hard work undertaken by the course team that had ensured successful implementation of the course was commented on favourably by the external examiners. They also commented on the excellent staff team spirit and the enthusiastic approach to education demonstrated by senior clinicians. These factors had made it possible to implement the course programme so effectively. The commitment to achieve high standards demonstrated by all staff involved with the course was recognised and again commented upon.[35]

The second cohort on the course completed their studies at the end of the 1992–3 academic year. There was a considerable spread of ability in this group, but, in the final assessment, twelve of the twenty members of the cohort had achieved distinction in the written papers, practical examination, assignment work or the clinical examination. In total, twenty-one distinctions were awarded over the four categories and a further four merits in the clinical examination. One candidate, Heather Vernon, was awarded distinction in all categories and a further five gained distinction in two categories. Staff considered that with such a spread of distinctions, it would be implied that the course assessment procedures had been applied with insufficient rigour. However, the external examiners reassured them that the assessment and marking had been of a high standard totally consistent with CSP requirements.

Once the course was completed, its advantages were considered to be:

- increased flexibility of the course due to complete organisation and implementation on site
- variety of testing methods used suited a higher proportion of candidates than had been satisfied by the methods used in the national examination system
- final clinical examination was more closely related to current clinical practice.

Prior to implementation, the principal had considered the additional workload of internalisation could not be supported from within such a small staff. In this she totally underestimated their dedication, commitment and abilities as they had maintained their high ideals, accepting the additional responsibilities with cheerfulness and enthusiasm. They commented that the disadvantages they perceived were:

- additional time commitment for the external examiners to liaise with the CSP and the school
- additional time required by staff to prepare and implement the internalised examinations

- allowing choice in the location of the final clinical examination produced an uneven spread of examination implementation.

Another benefit of implementation of the internalised course was recognised as it had enabled them to gain experience in a range of activities that would not have been possible had the national examinations continued. They could now evaluate courses dispassionately, had developed confidence in supporting their individual points of view, and had become competent and confident in report writing and also in verbal and written presentation to their immediate colleagues and the CSP external examiners. The team had developed and matured throughout the four years of implementation of this course and entered the university system competent in all aspects of course development, implementation and review. The participating experience with the internalised course had proved to be of immense value, as was summarised by one of the external examiners, who wrote:

> It should be recorded that the staff of the school have shown great commitment to their tasks and advanced the learning experiences of students to a broader and wider spectrum of competencies. The planned transfer to higher education will offer the staff well-deserved opportunities to further develop the graduate programme while sustaining the sound clinical base so essential in care programmes. Their achievements are to be commended.[36]

The school could not have achieved such a successful course implementation without the patience, tolerance, expertise, support and encouragement given by the external examiners. They were generous with their time, perceptive in their assessments and applauded the obvious efforts made by staff to satisfy student expectations and CSP requirements. The principal and staff recognised the benefits of the external examiner system and were grateful for the preparation the course presented for the school's transfer to the academic environment.

Notes

[1] Extracts from the minutes of the Emergency ONSSP Policy Committee meeting, 27 July 1987

[2] Extracts from the minutes of the ONSSP Education Committee meeting, 17 December 1986

[3] Extracts from the minutes of the ONSSP Education Committee meeting, 25 February 1987

[4] Extracts from the minutes of the ONSSP Policy Committee meeting, 15 May 1987

[5] Extracts from the minutes of the ONSSP Policy Committee meeting, 25 February 1987

[6] Extracts from the minutes of the ONSSP Policy Committee meeting, 27 November 1987

[7] Ibid

[8] Extracts from the minutes of the Emergency ONSSP Policy Committee meeting, 27 July 1987

[9] Ibid

[10] Lord Halsbury, *Report of the Committee of Inquiry into the Pay and Related Conditions of Service of the Professions Supplementary to Medicine*, 1975

[11] Extracts from reports of the CPSM Interim Inspection, 11–12 July 1983, and CPSM Quinquennial Inspection, October 1986

[12] Extracts from CSP letter, 23 November 1987

[13] Extracts from the minutes of the ONSSP Policy Committee meeting, 29 January 1988

[14] Extracts from the minutes of the ONSSP Policy Committee meeting, 14 April 1988

[15] Ibid

[16] Reference to letter received from CSP, 15 June 1988, ref: Submission to the V&R panel, 26 May 1988

[17] Extracts from letter from the CSP, 29 November 1988

[18] Recommendation 8.6.d of the West Midlands Regional Training Services Report on Physiotherapy Training, August 1988

[19] Extracts from letter from CPSM, 28 June 1989

[20] Extracts from letter from CSP, 1 August 1989

[21] Extracts from the minutes of the ONSSP Policy Committee meeting, 29 January 1988

[22] Ibid

[23] Ibid

[24] Extracts from the minutes of the ONSSP Policy Committee meting, 13 April 1989

[25] Extracts from the minutes of the ONSSP Policy Committee meeting, 6 July 1989

[26] Extracts from the minutes of the ONSSP Policy Committee meeting, 5 December 1989

[27] Ibid

[28] Ibid

[29] Extracts from the minutes of the ONSSP Policy Committee meeting, 3 October 1990

[30] Ibid

[31] Ibid

[32] Extracts from the Graduate Diploma Course Report, September 1990

[33] Ibid

[34] Extracts from the Graduate Diploma Course Report, November 1991

[35] Extracts from the Graduate Diploma Course Report, December 1992

[36] Extracts from the Graduate Diploma Course Report, August 1993

Chapter 16
BSc (Honours) Physiotherapy

At the close of the consultation period on its 1988 report,[1] the RTC considered if it was advisable to permit all WM schools to develop pre-registration degrees. Eighty per cent of the districts consulted had favoured the idea and two schools – Coventry and Wolverhampton – planned to start validated courses in autumn 1989.[2] However, one or two members of the RTC considered the other three programmes should remain at diploma level to allow choice for candidates. The Regional Physiotherapy Training and Education Committee (RPTEC) also debated the matter at its first two meetings held on 4 April and 5 July 1989, when numerous arguments were presented in favour of equivalence in the level of qualification from all schools within the region's remit. Clinical and teaching staffs of the ONSSP, ROH and QE schools considered that, if their courses remained at diploma level, recruitment of staff and students would decline significantly over the next few years, to the detriment of the quality of the programmes.

After a long discussion in the policy committee, the ONSSP registered with the RTC its intent to develop a degree course.[3] The principal and her line manager from NSHA, Steve Bloor, were charged with the responsibility of initiating the proposal with an appropriate institution. As two years had elapsed since earlier discussions had been suspended on publication of the RTC interim statement, it was decided that the course under discussion at that time was obsolete; negotiation of a totally new proposal was required. To this end, a letter and questionnaire were prepared and circulated to a number of institutions who might be interested in such a development. The letter invited a declaration of interest and the questionnaire requested detailed information about the validation procedure operated by the institution, the anticipated timescale for development and the facilities and staffing resources that could be allocated to the programme.

Four of the seven institutions contacted responded positively to the proposal. Chester College and Keele University referred to previous course development proposals with which they had been involved. Crewe and Alsager College and Wolverhampton Polytechnic also gave detailed positive responses to the questionnaire.[4] It was decided to investigate these four centres further and Kevin Gittings, the assistant treasurer of NSHA, and Ken Stopani, assistant principal of the school based in NSHA, joined Steve Bloor and the principal on visits to each centre for more detailed discussions. Analysis of the information gained from the visits determined that Keele University was the most appropriate location for course development.

Keele offered support in physics, psychology and physiology (to be taught by the biological science department) to accommodate the required twenty-five per cent of course teaching to be undertaken by the university when developing a degree course in conjunction with an external institution. To facilitate understanding of physiotherapy course requirements, representatives of the three departments concerned were invited to the Oswestry base of the school. A programme was arranged to demonstrate the range of subject matter covered by the syllabus, the level of teaching required to support current physiotherapy practice and the academic level of the existing student body. University representatives appreciated this input, commenting that the day was informative and enabled them to gain a firm understanding of the requirements of the new course. Following exploratory visits by the CSP director of education to the ONSSP and Keele University, the school was granted permission to proceed with course development.[5] Syllabi were realigned with apportionment of subject teaching to accommodate the university input to the course; the course outline presented to the V&R panel in November 1990 was accepted prior to preparation of full course documentation.[6]

Following this promising start, the university determined that it could not proceed with detailed planning until it was assured that the funding was secure. As the Health Authorities would not commit to funding the course until the content was finalised, a small impasse was reached.[7] Fortunately, this occurred only after completion of preliminary discussions, but retarded the proposed starting date of the course by a year.

Working Paper 10 was produced[8] about this time in which it was proposed that from April 1991, regions should plan to be self sufficient, training physiotherapists to satisfy their individual needs. It stated that financial responsibility for physiotherapy education should be transferred to the regions hosting schools and not borne by the Health Authorities in which the schools were based. The West Midlands region, recognised to overproduce physiotherapists, had yet to publish its response to Working Paper 10 when the university required assurance of the security of course funding. If it were to be developed on schedule, the Health Authorities concerned would have to guarantee financial support from their existing resources. They were concerned that the arrangements the WMRHA ultimately made could negate Working Paper 10's proposals, placing a continuing financial strain on the Health Authorities supporting the course.

Despite this uncertainty, the Health Authorities took the brave decision to support course development and held a series of meetings with the university to identify funding requirements. This was finalised by November when Dr Slade, Director of Academic Affairs at Keele University, determined the specific pricing model to be used to charge for the course, based on the University Funding Council's (UFC) guide price for students studying courses allied to medicine. The figure to be charged to the Health Authorities was reduced by acceptance that a number of services offered to full-time students, such as use of the library and social facilities, would not be required or would be utilised far less by the 'part-time' physiotherapy students. Student Union membership was already provided through CSP enrolment and a further reduction was offered in recognition of the anticipated contribution to university activities that would be made by ONSSP staff. This resulted in an annual tuition fee of £4,800/student with the Health Authorities being charged a twenty-five per cent share of this, £1,200.[9] Negotiators recognised the calculations presented a very fair costing of the university's contribution to the course and papers were sent to each Health Authority requesting confirmation of the financial support required to enable course development to continue. The detailed costing information was sent to the WMRHA in anticipation it would ultimately implement the proposals outlined by Working Paper 10 and assume financial responsibility for course support.

Additional costs of £20,000 were incurred by the Health Authorities for upgrading the school's IT and laboratory equipment to university standards. University records were already electronically based and both staff and undergraduates were expected to be computer literate in order to work and study effectively. At that time, the use of computers in individual hospital departments was yet to be realised. It was only after hard negotiation with the northern unit that the school was eventually permitted to purchase a single desktop computer and staff were able to achieve basic competence in its use before its transfer to the university campus.

The schedule for validation required preparation, printing and circulation of multiple copies of all relevant documents by a certain date. NSHA had prepared course documentation required for submission and subsequent validation events of the graduate diploma course, but was unable to continue this support for the degree and the costs of both course development and reproduction of the supportive documentation devolved to the northern unit SHA. All syllabus contributions were received within predetermined time limits and school staff completed course documentation to the standard and in the style and format required by the university. Steve Bloor, who had provided great enthusiasm, leadership and encouragement in the early stages of the proposal, facilitating selection of the location for this course development, unfortunately left the Health Authority before the project was completed.[10]

Development of the degree marked the climax of course reconstruction that had been an ongoing process throughout the 1980s. Since 1981, the school had received many benefits from the enlightened approach to course delivery introduced by the student teachers undertaking the Certificate in Education programme at Wolverhampton Polytechnic. Many had remained with the school after qualification and brought a dynamic and enthusiastic approach to syllabus teaching. Over the previous decade innovative and diverse course assessment procedures were developed and assimilated into the school's programme. Ken Stopani had spearheaded this development and, at the time of the initiation of the degree development discussions, the assessment procedures in place for the academic components of the internalised diploma course operated by the school required little modification or change to satisfy university criteria. Both school and university staff were confident that all professional aspirations and academic requirements for the degree course were satisfied and the definitive documentation was completed for the tripartite validation.

This first course produced by the two institutions was always to be a compromise due to the different backgrounds and development of the hosting institutions. The university as an autonomous institution had evolved a flexible, sophisticated academic and research culture that could be adapted to meet individual course requirements. Physiotherapy, by contrast, came from an educationally deprived background where the prime responsibility was the training of a skilled and competent workforce to meet clinical needs. Courses were funded by the NHS, operated to a national standard determined by the CSP, and approved and monitored by the CPSM. Approximately thirty hospital-based schools operated these highly structured, examination-based courses to this national standard. Cessation of the CSP national examination system from the 1989 intake had triggered significant educational development of courses in schools but few had as yet developed a research culture. Unstinting encouragement, guidance and support freely given to the school by university staff enabled the different philosophies of the two institutions to be blended and a viable course was produced in a matter of months. Throughout the preparation period, the school was carrying a staff vacancy following the departure of one of its more senior experienced teachers, operating the second year of the graduate diploma course with internalised assessment and the final year of the course supported by the CSP national examinations.

In line with CSP guidelines, Nigel Palastanga, assistant dean of the faculty of health sciences at Cardiff University, agreed to be an external examiner to the degree course until completion of his term of primary responsibility to the graduate diploma course. This was of great assistance as he had already gained knowledge of staff capabilities, strengths and weaknesses during his current involvement with the school.

Staff had gained considerable experience in course validation as a result of the protracted process of acceptance of the internalised course and approached the validation event on 7 June 1991 with confidence. At this event, attended by school staff, clinical educators and students, representatives from the university, the CPSM and CSP examined all aspects of the course presented to the meeting. The principal was able to report a successful outcome to the policy committee in July.[11] The draft report subsequently received from the validation team of the university commented favourably on the student-centred approach to teaching and considered the course appropriate for the modern needs of physiotherapy. They appeared very supportive of the school, were impressed by the personal development undertaken by all members of the teaching staff and indicated that teaching on the existing diploma course was of degree standard.[12]

Some 'minor' adjustments to the documentation were required before the privy council would grant final approval of the course. Clearly defined distinction between the graduate diploma course currently implemented by the school and the proposed honours degree course was requested and the development team was asked to review the final assessment qualifying examination with an increase in the weighting of the clinical competence and research components. Documentation was to be revised and illustrated with clear diagrams or flow charts with reconsideration of some of the academic course content to eliminate perceived overemphasis of subject input supportive of, but not immediately concerned with, the practice of physiotherapy. More detail of the proposed University Induction Programme was required and finally, transfer of 100 hours of the proposed clinical education programme to the research project was suggested to improve balance.[13]

This was a significant list for a course that had received a positive response to validation; however, the team required no substantive changes to the course presented and clear guidance had been given for the revisions requested. Ken Stopani undertook the task of revision and resubmitted the course on 16 August, several weeks ahead of the deadline. The CSP and CPSM accepted the new course documentation as presented and Keele University's validation and academic affairs committees re-examined the paperwork. No further objections were raised and formal approval of the course was granted for implementation to five cohorts, running out with the students due to graduate in 1998. This information was received during the first week in September, shortly before the arrival of the first cohort.[14] A major factor influencing the speed and efficacy of this course's acceptance was the absence of significant RTC activity during the preparation period and the course presented was considered on merit. The school was identified as an affiliated college of the university to enable staff use of university facilities to initiate independent research.[15]

It had been predicted that establishment of a degree programme would stimulate application to the course. This proved to be the case as the first cohort, recruited prior to course validation, was selected from an application pool of 220; the second and third cohorts, recruited following implementation of the degree, were selected from application pools of 590 and approximately 2,000 respectively. Following course validation, applications had increased significantly in both quality and quantity with considerable interest displayed by potential students with alternative sources of funding who would not be reliant on NHS bursary support. The university was encouraged by the popularity of the course, indicating it initially matched and subsequently exceeded the levels of interest attracted by courses in psychology, criminology and law, proven over the years to be the most popular courses offered by the university.

Twenty-three students were accepted to the first cohort, twenty supported by NHS bursaries and three privately funded (two from Brunei and one with Swedish entry qualifications).[16] The second cohort also numbered twenty-three, but only eighteen were supported by NHS bursaries and five were privately funded (two Norwegian, and one each from Scotland, Brunei and the United States). These students were generally satisfied with the course and commented that organisation was good, facilities adequate and the course demanding but enjoyable.[17] The third cohort was selected early in February 1993 when eighteen candidates supported by NHS bursaries and ten Norwegian students were offered places, predicting that the course cohort would number twenty-eight. For the first time, recruitment to the total authorised CPSM intake had been achieved, despite ten places not being funded by the NHS.

Transport was required to enable students to attend the university component of the course. At that time, RJAH owned a bus that was used to take patients and staff to local events. These journeys were significantly shorter than the journey to Keele and few problems were encountered. The bus was rapidly approaching the end of its useful life and there was concern that the regular commitment of approximately 200 miles a week would accelerate its demise. The first cohort, undertaking the journey throughout the winter months, complained of the cold and travel sickness due to unreliable and ineffective heating in the bus and the excessive vibration and fumes suffered when the engine was running. The bus broke down on three occasions and, on these days, students missed their university classes. Problems were also encountered in providing drivers owing to rationalisation of the transport department of the hospital with subsequent reduction in the numbers of drivers employed. It is reported that the students' travel arrangements were maintained only by the goodwill of individuals who accommodated the journeys during off-duty time. It was a most inefficient use of the driver's time as he was responsible for the transport of the students between hospital and university, but had no defined duties for the hours between the scheduled journeys. These problems were eliminated in the second year as a coach large enough to accommodate two sets of students was contracted from a local transport firm.[18] Once at the university, students followed a defined timetable, but when not actually in lectures they were without allocated space in which to relax or study, unlike full-time students who could return to their campus-based accommodation. During lunch breaks they could be found sitting on the floor lining the walls of the chancellor's building, surrounded by their belongings, obviously cold and miserable, as they attempted to eat lunch and raise enthusiasm for the afternoon's activities. With the arrival of the second cohort, students were observed to be much more at ease in the university environment; they had started to use the general campus facilities and were making good use of the university committee structure to voice their opinions.

Once the course started, school staff readjusted teaching schedules to accommodate seventy-five per cent of the total syllabus in sixty per cent of the teaching week that resulted from the time commitment to the university. The consequent reduction in the time available for practical subject teaching placed considerable additional pressures on accommodation use at the Oswestry base and it was determined that conversion of the Mary Powell Room from a theory to a practical room would facilitate timetabling. The purchase of additional plinths and storage of the desks that had previously furnished the room was eventually achieved with considerable ease of pressure on staff involved in the teaching of practical subjects.[19]

Although students enrolled for 1991 entry were delighted the course had been upgraded to a degree, they identified problems at each stage of course implementation that were addressed by staff and mostly remedied, substantially improving the university experience for the second and subsequent cohorts following the programme. Their comprehensive comments recorded in the annual course reviews covered transport problems, communication issues, styles of teaching, assessment procedures and correlation of subjects where responsibility was shared between the two institutions.

Some students initially found difficulty in coming to terms with the style of teaching used by the university, with resultant low motivation particularly in psychology, where an extensive syllabus was covered in great depth that had little application to health care needs.[20] This situation was reflected by the students' poor performance in the end-of-year assessments. On completion of the first year programme, the syllabus, assessment, communication and teaching methods were reviewed. The lecturer responsible for the course gained a better understanding of the physiotherapist's role and consequent student needs from the course by observational visits to various physiotherapy departments. This additional understanding, supported by regular interdepartmental meetings between school and university, substantially improved the course and student performance in subsequent end-of-year assessments.[21]

The physics department used a team teaching approach for this subject. Despite significant variation in the pre-course level of knowledge of individuals within the first cohort, a very high level of satisfaction was recorded, with any minor problems encountered relating to the appropriate pitch of lectures being immediately addressed. With standardised pre-entry knowledge and ability within subsequent groups, tutor satisfaction was much higher than with the first cohort and matched student perceptions. Physics teaching was coordinated with the electrotherapy syllabus taught by the school. This was considered effective for the first cohort; however, the explanations of the physiological effects of the modalities taught was hampered by the fact that the agreed teaching of inflammation changes by the biological science department had not occurred.[22] Unfortunately, the second cohort recorded an extremely high level of dissatisfaction with the electrotherapy course. Students commented that lectures lacked structure and relevance. They complained that the examination was not based on the teaching and failed to conform to published information regarding content and balance of questions. They found practical sessions to be badly organised and haphazard with inadequate instruction on machine use. Sessions were often unsupervised due to the unexplained absence of the tutor. The member of staff concerned unfortunately did not recognise the problems and only identified that the group was very keen and learned quickly.[23]

ONSSP staff taught the majority of the anatomy syllabus by directed student learning supported by tutorials, regular assessment and classes in surface and functional anatomy. Divided into 'packages' of learning, the course continued throughout the first year. With the reduction of time at the Oswestry base, the method of teaching this subject placed additional pressure and stress on students, particularly during the second term. Staff responded immediately to their comments, reviewed theoretical, practical and tutorial content of the course, introduced a lead lecture to give an overview and set out the priorities of each new 'package' and modified course assessment procedures. A rest week on completion of the lower limb prior to commencement of studies of the upper limb was introduced. Finally, the course in cadaveric anatomy negotiated for delivery by the Postgraduate School of Medicine at Stoke-on-Trent and the Institute of Orthopaedics at Oswestry was discontinued as it was no longer required by the CSP curriculum of study.[24] These measures greatly improved the loading of the course for the second and subsequent cohorts.

The most significant problems were encountered with the teaching of physiology as this subject had been divided and apportioned between the two institutions. It soon became obvious that there were areas of the syllabus agreed for university delivery that were not being covered, with duplication of other components. Laboratory work was hampered by the late delivery of, and failures in, the working of equipment ordered for the purpose. As the published physiology syllabus was required in its entirety to facilitate understanding of the effects of physiotherapeutic interventions students would implement during the clinical component of the course, this was a major problem. Appointment of a lecturer to support the students' specific needs during the second term and frequent additional meetings between school and university were hoped to improve the situation.[25] However, despite many consultations with the department and monitoring of the course by school staff, university teaching of this subject continued to give rise to concern. Cell biology overlapped significantly with the A-level biology syllabus and subsequently students holding this qualification were exempted from the course. As A-level biology was a condition of entry for school leavers, the decision relieved some pressure on the second and subsequent cohorts while giving mature students the opportunity to gain essential knowledge in this area. The second cohort commented they found the genetics course, now concentrating on human genetics, very interesting but, unfortunately, this was not the case of the teaching of cardiovascular physiology. Students complained that lectures continued to be disorganised and had little focus, a situation confirmed by the school member of staff who monitored this area. By contrast, laboratory work was much improved with the sessions being well structured and supervised. This was greatly facilitated by team teaching with a teacher from the school who was able to monitor content and explain relevance to both university colleagues and students.

ONSSP staff taught the remaining curricular subjects either independently or with maintenance of existing collaborative links with other departments such as ORLAU. In these areas, all course objectives were met for the first cohort, with high or very high levels of satisfaction recorded by the student body.[26] This was to be expected as the staff involved were experienced in the areas of their responsibilities and were competent in coordinating their subject areas with the rest of the physiotherapy curriculum. With the exception of electrotherapy theory and practice, all subjects that were the responsibility of the school to deliver to the second and subsequent cohorts achieved their objectives and continued to be awarded high or very high student satisfaction ratings. Problems identified with regard to electrotherapy teaching were, unfortunately, not resolved.

The Part 1 examination had been expanded to include additional papers in physiology, behavioural science and the scientific bases of physiotherapeutics to accommodate the subjects taught by the university. ONSSP took responsibility for the anatomy papers and viva, the OSPE examination and coordinated the scientific bases of physiotherapeutics paper between the ONSSP, ORLAU and the physics department of the university. The university was responsible for physiology and psychology papers. Students were also required by the university to complete set coursework in psychology and physiology. It was apparent that, whereas both institutions recognised the importance of the first-year examinations as a hurdle to pass before continuance of the course, there was a different emphasis on their importance. Physiotherapy used a highly structured assessment system placing equal importance to all examinations held throughout the course, whereas the university placed more emphasis on those held in years two and three that contributed to the classification of the degree.

Early problems arose with the circulation of examination papers for review by the external examiners. Whereas ONSSP staff had prepared these many months in advance of requirement, university staff had a far more relaxed approach. The external examiner was particularly concerned that he did not receive papers from the psychology or biological science departments in time to evaluate them effectively or implement any required modifications. He made several recommendations for improvements in the conduct of the first-year assessment programme that required immediate attention. As a meeting organised in November 1992 to address the problems was attended by only one representative from the university, the situation remained unresolved for the second cohort.[27]

The university used a pass mark of forty per cent for all examination components including coursework, whereas the school required the achievement of fifty-five per cent to pass a paper and sixty per cent to succeed in a practical examination. First year examinations were taken by twenty-one of the first cohort and, of these, thirteen passed at the first attempt and two delayed entry on health grounds. These results were in line with university experience, but, owing to the different emphasis placed on the examination by the two institutions, lack of success was handled differently. The university had a more flexible approach than the school, which offered automatic retake of failed components as the only option. The university offered this opportunity, but in some instances students were required to resubmit coursework as an alternative or in addition to retaking the examination. Also, one of the students who had delayed entry on health grounds was exempted totally from the physiology examination by virtue of having completed coursework to a satisfactory level.[28] However, all students were eventually successful and entered the second year of the course on schedule. The first year examination results for the second cohort reflected the efforts undertaken to fine-tune the course, improve communication, cope with the split site and become more comfortable with defined roles and responsibilities. Of the twenty-three entrants to the examination, twenty-two passed all components at the first attempt. The unsuccessful candidate continued to the second year having resubmitted coursework in biological sciences and successfully retaken examinations in biological sciences, psychology and anatomy.

Nigel Palastanga, the external examiner, considered the course had gone well during its first year of implementation and congratulated staff on the standards achieved. He made several recommendations for improvement, particularly in biological science and with regard to the university examination regulations. His recommendations were all addressed and diligently pursued prior to the arrival of the second cohort in autumn 1992.

The university appointed external examiners as the course entered its second year. University statutes dictate that they should be of professorial grade and, at the time, there were only two professors of physiotherapy in the UK, one with a research background and one based in education. Professor Sandra Myles had been involved with implementation of the first degree course in physiotherapy developed on the UK mainland at Queens College, Glasgow. Being of the appropriate status and having exemplary educational expertise, she was approached and appointed external examiner to the course to act on behalf of the university. Nigel Palastanga, who was now dean of the faculty of health sciences at Cardiff, was already in post and Simon Mockett, a senior teacher from Nottingham School of Physiotherapy, was appointed to the third position. The school was confident that these appointments brought the most highly qualified and experienced people available to support the course. The individuals concerned were of sufficient standing to satisfy the university and with their experience of physiotherapy degree courses they could guide ONSSP staff to implement the course at the appropriate level to meet all university, CPSM and CSP criteria.

The start of the 1992 academic year brought further change as the university introduced semesterisation to replace the three-term academic year. Initially, there was little course realignment required as the revised schedules and timings affected only the university components and could be accommodated without disruption to the teaching input. The overall length of the year was not affected so there was no requirement for significant rearrangement of teaching schedules.[29]

The most significant aspect of the second-year course was the start of the two-year clinical education programme. The major variation from earlier courses operated by the school was the introduction of assessed student performance on each clinical placement. Placement assessment graded student performance and awarded a mark that would contribute to the final award and classification of honours received by the student on course completion. This was a welcome innovation, recognising the educational role of clinical exposure rather than viewing it as a training requirement.

Students were very satisfied with the new arrangements, and the level of supervision and instruction they received in clinical areas, and they considered the scheduled liaison visits by academic tutors to be of great value. The three-day week, necessitated by university commitments, was not satisfactory as it reduced the experience, learning opportunities and students' perceptions of involvement with the continuity of departmental activity. Clinical educators, who had adopted the new procedures with enthusiasm, commented positively on the motivation, level of interest and eagerness to learn displayed by the majority of the students.[30]

Second-year university studies produced higher levels of satisfaction than had been reported by students during the previous year. In behavioural science, they were introduced to counselling and psychotherapy, research appreciation and measurement theory in physiotherapy. Course objectives were met, but there were difficulties in timetabling and workload that produced high levels of stress and some absenteeism. Students gained a good overall introduction to research methodology with lectures supported by tutorials. Realising the importance of this area to support third-year studies, they would have appreciated increased input on statistics and clearer guidance for writing assignments. They expressed disappointment that bereavement and the grieving process was not covered in the counselling course although it had been specifically requested – a situation that was remedied for subsequent cohorts. The neuroscience department of the university taught neurology and neuropathology, with the physiotherapeutic management of neurological conditions covered by ONSSP staff. Owing to the reduction of hours available for ONSSP teaching in this area, emphasis was placed on the neurological conditions most likely to be met by students on clinical placement. Guided reading lists were distributed to augment knowledge of neurological conditions not covered in detail, but this was not wholly satisfactory.[31] As before, the professional areas of the course implemented by ONSSP were well received and students accepted that the readjustment of the programme for the management of neurological conditions had been necessary and commented that it prepared them adequately for early placement in this area.

During the year the external examiners diligently scrutinised all aspects of the programme on behalf of the university and CPSM, and wrote detailed assessment reports. They applauded the manner in which staff had overcome problems of the split site, set a high standard on the course, coped well with uncertainty about the school's future and responded positively to address recommendations made the previous year.[32]

The clinical education component of the course was progressing well; high standards and effective communication between school and hospital had been maintained throughout. External examiners commented that the school team and clinical staff had obviously worked closely together to develop an assessment tool that was workable, interpretable and fair. Students were confident with all aspects of the course and clearly understood and had confidence in the assessment instrument.[33]

Major criticisms were levelled against the organisation and implementation of the course assessment programme. Course regulations were not comprehensive and were open to misinterpretation. Also the schedule for assessment was unclear and the administration of assessment needed attention.[34] The criticism of the situation was not levelled against school staff, but reflected the lack of leadership given by the university in this area. The university was instructed immediately to give the school a full set of their appropriate documentation to enable the 'competent team' to construct a set of course-specific regulations that would be pertinent to all elements and servicing departments of the course. The school was also required to develop and circulate an assessment calendar to ensure that all material submitted could be scrutinised by the external examiners in time for constructive criticism and advice to be acted upon.[35]

The external examiners' comments and criticisms finally persuaded the university to produce the University of Keele Selected Ordinances, Regulations and Examination Information, which should have been made available prior to course validation. ONSSP staff adapted and incorporated this information into the much-needed course-specific regulations that were approved by the university and CPSM and subsequently circulated to all parties involved with the course. Production of this document largely eliminated the persistent and justified complaints made by students, staff and examiners regarding the course assessment procedures, allowing improved course appreciation.

External examiners were very concerned that the level of course assessment was not fit for purpose. A three-year vocational honours degree should, from the outset, present students with the opportunity for discursive, analytical and evaluative expression; they commented that only the psychology paper was pitched at the appropriate level.[36] If papers had been submitted in accordance with the normal time schedule, necessary improvements would have been proposed to lift them to honours degree level, enabling students to demonstrate their full capabilities. However, the papers had, for a second year, been submitted too late to allow substantive changes to be made. University guidance in the level of assessment required was urgently needed to help the team, who had no previous experience in this area, to develop a style of examination that was discriminatory and allowed demonstration and reward for higher levels of learning. Continuing inaction by the university had placed the course in jeopardy and was not to be allowed to continue for a third year.[37] Students had performed well in the examinations set, but, as these required only lower levels of learning, such as factual recall, they were not able to demonstrate their abilities fully.

The most significant problem that had arisen due to the absence of comprehensive course regulations was the level of guidance and support given to second-year students to help them prepare effectively for the presentation of the research project in the third year. With preparation and acceptance of comprehensive course regulations by the start of the third year and a high level of tutorial support by staff of the departments in which their projects were set, the situation was somewhat redeemed. That they all submitted on time and satisfied university requirements is more a testament to their ability, dedication and determination to succeed than to the efficacy of course organisation.

They were the first cohort to graduate, having completed their studies in June 1994. A very articulate group, they had readily ascribed to the course evaluation procedures and had been fair in their assessments across the range of activities reviewed. Their comments enabled necessary improvements to be made at each stage of the course and they also predicted potential problem areas, enabling staff to act before these affected course implementation. They graduated from the university in December 1994 at a ceremony attended by parents, friends and staff involved with the course. ONSSP staff were honoured to be invited to participate in the proceedings but were surprised and a little disconcerted on this occasion to be filtered out from the academic procession and made to sit in the front row of the auditorium rather than continuing to the platform. It was obvious that the university did not yet recognise physiotherapy as a university-based academic subject worthy of equal consideration to traditional campus departments. Graduate entry to physiotherapy was finally achieved in 1994 and the first to qualify from the course operated by Keele University and the ONSSP were part of this major progression in level of professional entry qualification. They were followed a year later by the second cohort who were, as it happens, the last to complete the programme, although approval had been granted initially for a further three cohorts.

Notes

[1] West Midlands Regional Training Services (Training and Education Section) Report on Physiotherapy Training in the West Midlands Region, August 1988

[2] WMRHA RTC meeting, 20 February 1989

[3] Extracts from the minutes of the ONSSP Policy Committee meeting, 6 July 1989

[4] Extracts from the minutes of the ONSSP Policy Committee meeting, 15 December 1989

[5] Extracts from the minutes of the ONSSP Policy Committee meeting, 28 June 1990

[6] Extracts from the minutes of the ONSSP Policy Committee meeting, 3 October 1990

[7] Extracts from the minutes of the Policy Committee meeting, 28 June 1990

[8] 'Working for Patients – Education and Training in the NHS' (further guidance), 1989

[9] Extracts from letter dated 30 November 1990 from Dr Slade to the principal of ONSSP

[10] Extracts from the minutes of the ONSSP Policy Committee meeting, 28 June 1990

[11] Extracts from the minutes of the ONSSP Policy Committee meeting, 1 July 1991

[12] Ibid

[13] Ibid

[14] Extracts from the minutes of the ONSSP Policy Committee meeting, 9 October 1991

[15] Extracts from the minutes of the ONSSP Policy Committee meeting, 1 July 1991

[16] Extracts from the BSc (Hons) Course Report, July 1992

[17] Extracts from the BSc (Hons) Course Report, August 1993

[18] Extracts from the minutes of the ONSSP School Management Board meeting, 17 August 1992

[19] Ibid

[20] Extracts from the BSc (Hons) Course Report, July 1992.

[21] Extracts from the BSc (Hons) Course Report, August 1993

[22] Extracts from the BSc (Hons) Course Report, July 1992

[23] Extracts from the BSc (Hons) Course Report, August 1993

[24] Extracts from the BSc (Hons) Course Report, July 1992

[25] Extracts from the BSc (Hons) Course Report, July 1992, and from the minutes of the ONSSP School Management Board meeting, 17 August 1992

[26] Extracts from the BSc (Hons) Course Report, July 1992

[27] Extracts from the BSc (Hons) Course Report, August 1993

[28] Extracts from the BSc (Hons) Course Report, July 1992

[29] Extracts from the minutes of the ONSSP School Management Board meeting, 5 October 1992

[30] Extracts from the BSc (Hons) Course Report, August 1993

[31] Ibid

[32] Ibid

[33] Ibid

[34] Ibid

[35] Ibid

[36] Ibid

[37] Ibid

Chapter 17
Rationalisation of Schools of Physiotherapy in the West Midlands Region

Proposals to reduce the number of physiotherapy courses in the West Midlands region were originally presented in the late 1960s by the CSP and CPSM. However, following extensive discussion with the RHA, not one of the several proposals submitted was pursued, owing to the region's inability to determine the most appropriate way forward and the predicted implementation costs of each suggestion.[1] Twenty years later, following several attempts to achieve such reduction, recommendations contained in Working Paper 10[2] brought matters to a head. It was proposed, in this paper, that from April 1991 financial responsibility for physiotherapy education should be borne by the regions hosting schools and not by the Health Authorities in which schools were based. The WMRHA made no definitive response to the paper by its scheduled implementation date and two months after this the joint KU/ONSSP degree course was validated. Shropshire and North Staffordshire Health Authorities enabled this achievement by funding the development and guaranteeing financial support for initial implementation of the course from their own resources.

There was a significant national shortage of physiotherapists working in the NHS during the late eighties and early nineties. All schools of physiotherapy were encouraged to recruit to their total CPSM-validated entry numbers in 1992 to improve the supply of qualified staff in the medium term to address this shortfall. The West Midland region was severely affected by the shortages and had reduced services in several clinical areas. However, WMRHA responded to this national request by introducing a ten per cent reduction in the numbers of bursary-funded places to all schools within its remit. Despite the high level of national and regional vacancies, the region remained concerned that it was training more physiotherapists than required to maintain its workforce and offered its 'spare' capacity to regions who were under-training, proposing they sponsored students to West Midlands schools. The outcome of these discussions was disappointing with little sponsorship being achieved.

To ensure implementation of its subsequent plans, the region had first to eliminate the opportunity for individual schools, notably the ONSSP, to challenge future rationalisation proposals and to this end, in November 1991, it circulated direction for the establishment of committee structures that would make schools directly accountable to the region. Through the new organisational relationships, the region proposed to contract for education provision directly with the schools.[3] Local general managers were to act on behalf of the hosting Health Authorities and Gordon Braid of the northern unit SHA was nominated to negotiate on behalf of the ONSSP, supported by a small management board. Membership of the one determined for the ONSSP was Kirk MacKenzie, deputy director of personnel for NSHA, Gordon Braid, general manager of the northern unit of SHA, Ron Parry, assistant UGM (finance) of the northern unit of SHA and the principal.[4] In addition, there was to be an education committee with representation from all providers of, and participants in, the programme provided by the school. A staff/student liaison committee completed the triad of the committee structure required by the region and replaced the ONSSP policy committee in June 1992.

On 1 November 1991 a meeting was held between the RPTEC purchasing team and administrative staff from SHA and NSHA representing the ONSSP to determine the school contract for the following year. At this meeting, the region identified a raft of proposals, initiating its response to Working Paper 10. The first of these was the reduction of the number of allocated NHS-funded bursaries for the school from twenty to eighteen for the 1992 intake. The last quinquennial inspection by CPSM/CSP in 1986 recommended the award of twenty-eight bursaries annually, a level of funding never implemented owing to the financial constraints of the funding Health Authorities.[5] In mild contradiction to the reduction of funded bursary places, school operational costs for 1992/1993 were to be calculated on the basis of acceptance of a cohort of twenty to enable retention of existing staff and maintain staff–student ratios. The recruitment of additional students not eligible for bursary support was permissible. Although the funding level for the year was to be based on the existing funded staff/student ratios, there was no guarantee offered for the support of subsequent intakes to the school. The school was now in a very vulnerable position and this reduction in bursary places was considered by many to be the first step in its ultimate closure. As it was also announced at the meeting that there was to be a further comprehensive review of physiotherapy education provision in the West Midlands with publication of a definitive final report in June–July 1992, there was little scope for optimism.[6]

SHA and NSHA were expected to bear the costs of development and initial implementation of the degree course but the region agreed to support annual recurring costs arising from the development. This was a very disappointing result for the Health Authorities, who had so generously supported the development in the hopes that WMRHA would reimburse their financial outlay when recommendations contained in Working Paper 10 were implemented.[7] Finally, at this meeting, the region withdrew sponsorship for the potential student teacher who expected to be accepted to the 1992 Wolverhampton course. The school was unable to pursue the application it had received as the region placed an embargo on all training of teachers until the outcome of the latest review was known.

Following many concerns raised by the schools regarding the accuracy of statistics presented in earlier reports to which they had no input, a moderate change to working arrangements was announced. School principals were to meet regularly with nominated regional representatives to present accurate factual and statistical information about the operation of their courses and staffing issues. Schools were again subjected to scrutiny by an evaluation team and, although an extensive written submission was required to support the ONSSP visit in March 1992, its purpose was never clearly defined.[8] The visit unsettled and concerned staff, who had been subjected to abnormal stresses and considerable pressure for a number of years due to RTC activity, necessary course development and continuing commitment to the courses operated by the school.

Questions were raised about future funding and organisation of clinical education programmes following transfer of managerial and financial accountability of schools to the region. With unitisation of clinical budgets, particularly in Shropshire, it was becoming increasingly difficult to maintain existing arrangements.[9] The region had not yet considered this aspect of course maintenance but determined that there would be no change to the existing arrangements and clinical education should continue to be funded by districts. They referred immediate concerns to the general managers now responsible for negotiating the annual contracts. It was stated the academic institutions hosting degree courses were not expected to be responsible for funding clinical education, only staff travel incurred supporting the programmes and student transport to placements. Course leaders queried how these arrangements would affect the maintenance and development of programmes but, as expected, received no response to their concerns.[10]

Although the contents of the proposed report remained undisclosed, schools were repeatedly assured that the recommendations drafted were based on actual evidence submitted and that the participants in the preparatory process would not be disconcerted by the contents of the final report scheduled for publication in July 1992. However, true to form, on the due date, an interim report only was published with the final report delayed until mid-September. The interim report requested information from the academic institutions hosting physiotherapy degrees concerning their plans for integration of the courses. However, it appears Coventry was not approached so submitted no response, whereas Wolverhampton and Keele submitted detailed proposals for full integration of their courses by autumn 1993. Birmingham University, which had not as yet undertaken any physiotherapy course development, was invited informally to submit a proposal but is thought to have declined due to the problems in the south of the city resulting from the proposed amalgamation of health districts in which the schools of physiotherapy were located.[11] By mid-September, the RHA was still not in a position to make a final decision and delayed publication of the report until the end of the year. At this stage, all four academic institutions in the region were invited to submit firm tenders for provision of their courses by 1994 and Keele updated its original submission.

The additional delay produced further complications for the school as Alan Stedman replaced Gordon Braid as UGM of the northern unit SHA in October 1992 and, at the same meeting, Mr Parry, the finance officer, announced his departure from the unit and indicated there were no plans to replace him.[12] Yet again, the school was left without access to informed financial information and advice at a critical time when the region was making many requests for detailed responses that were not within the purview of the staff to satisfy.

The CSP was extremely concerned about the continuation of the protracted review process as it could foresee potential disaster for the future of physiotherapy education in the region. Their concerns were raised and discussed with Sue Cox, WMRHA professional development manager, the Minister for Health, Virginia Bottomley, and George Blair from NHSME. The situation was subsequently monitored by these external agencies.[13]

A telephone call was received on 8 December from Sue Cox imparting the news that the report was ready for circulation. However, there was to be a further slight delay while the recommendations were presented to the RHA with subsequent publication of the definitive report before Christmas. Sue Cox stated that the region had readily made its decisions based on the evidence submitted and the delay in publication would have no impact on the content of the report nor the recommendations already determined.

By the third week in December the situation had changed and the last shred of confidence in the integrity of the review process evaporated. What had been a clear-cut decision, easily made, had developed into an extremely challenging and difficult situation that required further consideration. A new publication date of January 1993 was proposed for the report.[14] This further delay was of great concern to admissions tutors as the region had forbidden schools to make offers for the 1993 entry until their recommendations were known.

In January 1993 when the publication date was retarded yet again, schools were offered the choice between immediate award of bursaries for the 1993 entry on the basis of the 1992 allocations, or negotiation of bursary numbers at a later date when the RHA's decision would be known. As offers had to be made during February, schools opted for the first choice and in the second week of that month the ONSSP was allocated eighteen bursaries. By that time, the number of applications received for the course exceeded 1,700.[15] Wolverhampton and the ONSSP were subjected to another round of detailed investigation. Unfortunately, the production of the financial and statistical information required to support these visits was significantly hampered as the new UGM had little knowledge of physiotherapy education or the school and the unit had yet to appoint a finance officer to replace Mr Parry.

The long awaited, much delayed results of the review were received by fax on 18 March 1993 following acceptance of the recommendations by the RHA earlier in the day. No report was published then or later; however, a subsequent letter confirmed the result. It came as no surprise that the overall number of schools was to be reduced as this had been heralded throughout the consultation period. How this was to be achieved was disappointing as yet again recommendations made conflicted with the evidence submitted. The Royal Orthopaedic Hospital school was to merge with the Queen Elizabeth school and the combined school was to develop a degree with Birmingham University. Coventry school was to integrate with its host university and Wolverhampton school was to close. Finally, a fully integrated school of physiotherapy under university management was to be established on Keele campus by September 1994. The region had maintained its promise to reduce the numbers of schools in the region by amalgamation of the two Birmingham-based schools and closure of the Wolverhampton school. Once again, despite repeated advance assurances to the contrary, a politicised decision had been made that did not reflect the evidence submitted. The process that determined closure of one of the more successful schools in the region marred significantly the relief and pleasure in the ONSSP's ultimate success.

All staff employed and undergraduates enrolled on the KU/ONSSP BSc (Hons) course were to transfer to the new department.[16] Acceptance of the recommendation for closure of the ONSSP school base at midnight on the day selected for the move and the opening of the new hosting department on campus at 00.01 finally authorised the school to transfer to the university environment.

Once the final decision had been made, a schedule for implementation of the recommendations was determined. The region agreed to honour Wolverhampton school's commitment to the 1993 entry, the last cohort to be accepted by the school, and the Birmingham schools were to determine their own time schedule for course amalgamation and development of a degree programme. Evaluation of staffing levels in the remaining schools increased the ONSSP's establishment by two teachers, with the proviso that these additional staff appointments were to be made from within the region to protect staff displaced by the realignment of the schools.[17]

The ONSSP naively expected the transfer to the campus to be effected smoothly and efficiently, but this was not to be the case. The RTC had proposed this should occur by September/October 1994; however, in a letter received from the northern unit UGM the school was informed that agreement had been reached in principle with the university to advance the move by a year if it proved to be practical.[18]

On 30 April at a preliminary meeting to discuss issues appertaining to the transfer, Dr Slade identified that a bid by a commercial firm to provide the space quoted in the university tenders to the RHA was to be decided upon on 21 May. This was for the erection of a new department to house physiotherapy, radiography and nursing, planned for occupation by September 1993 – the preferred date agreed by Alan Stedman and Dr Slade for the school's transfer. However, the decision was not made on the expected date and, despite continued reassurance by the university, the possibility of building completion by September was unrealistic.

Possible locations for temporary teaching and office accommodation were identified in the biological science department and Keele Hall. Permission to evaluate this 'entirely suitable' accommodation was refused as Dr Slade considered it inappropriate to cause concern to the biological science department over the possible loss of teaching space that might not be required. He also indicated that the university would find it difficult but not impossible to complete the necessary alterations to the temporary facilities by September 1993. This subsumed the accommodation would meet CSP, CPSM, RHA and school requirements, and highlighted concern in the absence of opportunity for informed evaluation of the selected areas. Having agreed the tender conditions for course operation, the RHA refused to provide additional funding to support the conversion of space to temporary accommodation but, even as late as July, the university was assuring all parties that completion of the proposed building in Science Park 111 was certain for September 1993.

The next blow to the university's plans was the loss of the contract for the provision of radiography undergraduate education following a further RTC report recommending reduction of the number of regional schools of radiography from two to one. Totally new proposals for the housing of the School of Physiotherapy were required and the transfer date returned to autumn 1994.

The appropriate transfer of staff was an area for considerable negotiation and debate. The university was reluctant to respond to initial requests for information concerning salary and terms and conditions of employment as it was awaiting advice from the RHA concerning EC legislation on transferable rights of staff. These arrangements, the Transfer of Undertakings of Employment regulations, were collectively known by the acronym TUPE and were established to protect staff on transfer of courses to university or polytechnic bases from (in this instance) the NHS environment. The recommendations had not yet been tested as it appeared the ONSSP was to be the first school of physiotherapy to make use of them. Also, as the NSHA School of Nursing and Midwifery was making a line-by-line comparison of the rights and conditions of service between the NHS and the education sector, it was not considered appropriate for the ONSSP to 'reinvent the wheel'. A copy of the terms and conditions of employment for tutorial and administrative staff in universities was finally forwarded to the school on 3 June and planning of the staff appointment process was initiated.

The appointment of the head of department to manage the transfer of the school from the RJAH to the university campus was the first post to be determined. From the outset of the planning process, Sue Cox discouraged the current ONSSP principal from applying, indicating that the region expected her to retire now the school's future was secure. Having ascertained the most capable candidate for the post would be selected, the principal ignored the advice given and proceeded with an application. The only criterion that had been determined was that applicants should already be working in West Midlands schools. Applications for the post were received from Maggie Bailey (a senior teacher from Wolverhampton), Ken Stopani (assistant principal from the ONSSP) and Marian Tidswell (principal of the ONSSP). These candidates were interviewed in July by a panel consisting of Sue Cox (WMRHA professional development manager), Dr Slade (director of academic affairs from Keele University), Alan Stedman (representing the management board of the ONSSP) and the CSP advisor, Ian Rutherford (principal of the Nottingham School of Physiotherapy). The incumbent principal, Marian Tidswell, was offered the post during the afternoon when the interview panel had dispersed. In a break from normal procedure she was offered the post by the UGM who came to the school to impart the news personally and demanded immediate acceptance or rejection of the 'package' offered.

The conditions of the offer were quite punitive and reflected the RHA's reluctance to offer her the post. It was determined that if she accepted the offer, she would not be assimilated with the academic staff of the university, but would be seconded from the NHS to effect the transfer. The post was to be identified as the NHS management grade that most closely matched her current salary on the Whitley grade, Principal 111. Conditions of service associated with this new post offered an annual financial incentive bonus on salary in respect of change and improvements implemented by the department during the previous year. In this case, the base year was to be established as the next complete financial year, 1994/1995 with subsequent evaluation of the eligibility for the bonus based on year-on-year activity after that date. The first year of eligibility for the award was 1995/1996. By that time the school would be settled on campus, having completed more than a decade of significant change. Removal from the Principal 111 post denied the appointee further salary increases awarded to her existing post by the Whitley agreements. This proved to have a significant negative effect not only on salary received during the remaining years of employment, but also caused a quantitative reduction in the pension she was awarded on retirement.

Only a fool would accept a 'promotion' post that attracted such difficult working arrangements and negative financial conditions. Now that the school's future was secure, acceptance of the appointment would enable her to complete the project, even though she was to be denied the possibility of benefiting from the move to the education sector. In the final analysis, she did not have the courage to refuse the offer and, in accepting the post, probably made the biggest mistake of her career. With extreme reluctance, she accepted the terms, was appointed head of department and prepared to move the school from its NHS bases to the DoE environment.

This appointment effectively marked the end of the school's dependence on the NHS for financial and administrative support, and the remainder of the time at the hospital was concerned mainly with arrangements for the transfer to the university with the minimal disruption to staff and students. Marian, the last principal, had occupied the post for more than twelve years and had led the school through a time of significant change and development. The first five years of her tenure had been pleasurably concerned with the complete reorganisation of the school and its course to ensure that it met CPSM/CSP standards. She had been assisted significantly by the two funding Health Authorities, a very supportive sector administrator who was also secretary of the education committee of the school, her line manager in SHA and the League of Friends of the Robert Jones and Agnes Hunt Orthopaedic Hospital.

By October 1986, the time of the quinquennial review, the school was deemed to meet all statutory and professional requirements, all previously imposed restrictions were lifted and the future was bright. Unfortunately, less than six months after this inspection, when, ironically, there had been no gains or losses in either the staff or student populations, the Physiotherapy Evaluation Group of the Regional Training Council decided that the school was not educationally viable and announced it should be closed. This was patently untrue as the announcement was made following completion of the examination schedule. When the results of the national examinations were announced, both groups from the school led the field by substantial percentages and the regional health authority, with extreme reluctance, was forced to change its mind. After several more attempts to close the school either on its own or partnered in turn with Coventry, the Royal Orthopaedic School and Wolverhampton, it emerged in 1993 as one of the three schools in the region to transfer to the education sector.

During her tenure of post, Marian had been able to support twelve student teachers. Two had already gained qualification as teachers in secondary schools and followed the two-term professional course, joining the staff on qualification. The other ten undertook the course operated by the CSP at that time. One withdrew from the course before qualification returning to clinical work and seven of the remaining nine course qualifiers remained on the teaching staff for at least a year. One of the factors that assisted recruitment of so many teachers of such quality was the retention of the training budget, which enabled all staff to pursue master's courses. By the time of the transfer, all but one of the staff moving to the university had achieved a master's degree in a subject of choice that included ergonomics, habilitation, education and medical ethics. One member of staff was in the third year of a master's course by distance learning and one had already enrolled for a PhD. By 1994, the staff of the ONSSP were the most highly qualified in the country and well able to accept the academic opportunities offered by the university.

The course was initially supported by the CSP national examination system but, in 1989, a new course with internal assessment was introduced and two years later, the first degree course started in partnership with Keele University. Now Marian faced the final challenge of secondment from the NHS to transfer the course to the university campus.

The 1993 cohort for the Keele/ONSSP course had been agreed early in February of that year with eighteen candidates supported by NHS bursaries. Ten privately funded students were offered places, predicting that the course cohort would number twenty-eight. In July 1993, the Wolverhampton school decided to cancel its September intake and the ONSSP was awarded five additional bursaries to support candidates offered places by that school. On publication of the A-level results, the university was found to have recruited eight candidates above the bursary allocation and the ONSSP was faced with potential cohort of forty-eight, twenty above its CPSM/CSP approved numbers.

Representation was made immediately to the CPSM and CSP to allow the course to take the increased numbers and the WMRHA was asked to extend the bursary allocation for that year to accommodate the overshoot. Accommodation in the staff residency at RJAH was stretched to the limit, but the hospital was able to provide rooms for all students who wished to be resident. Theory-dedicated rooms could not accommodate the proposed increased numbers and use of the Institute of Orthopaedics lecture theatre and the staff training suite was arranged to solve the problem. Practical rooms in the school could accommodate a maximum of nineteen students to comply with CSP regulations and the solution in this case was to teach these subjects to a third of the cohort, repeating each practical session three times. Staff agreed to accept the additional teaching responsibilities and the CPSM, CSP and WMRHA gave their support on a one-off basis with dire warnings that they would be less sympathetic if the situation was repeated the following year.[19] Clinical education was scheduled to start in the second year of the course and it was considered that there would be ample time available to negotiate the additional placements required before the scheduled start of this aspect of the course.

Having settled the head of department post, recruitment of the remainder of the staff occurred in October. Senior posts available were aligned to reflect university responsibilities with appropriate job descriptions and people specifications prepared and circulated throughout the region. As a result of the interview process, Maggie Bailey, from the Wolverhampton school, was appointed to initiate departmental research and Sandy Robertson, from the Royal Orthopaedic Hospital school in Birmingham, accepted the post of admissions tutor. They both came to the ONSSP in February 1994 on release from their current posts. Marilyn Place was appointed course leader and Ken Stopani examinations officer. All remaining ONSSP staff who wished to transfer applied for and were appointed to lecturer posts. Determined that staff appointments would be made in accordance with the spirit of TUPE recommendations, the newly appointed head of department insisted that the university agreed to assimilate the staff appointed on to the appropriate academic structure on transfer to the university. This was agreed, but was difficult to implement. Subsequently, the directors of human resources based at the RJAH and Keele University and a senior Industrial Relations officer from the CSP were involved in difficult complex negotiations that extended over many months to ensure appropriate protection of the rights of these staff involved in the transfer.

Loss of the contract for radiography education forced the university to develop an alternative plan for the provision of suitable permanent accommodation for the school and a revised proposal was put out to tender. Delay in acceptance of the tender resulted from the proposal to build around a large protected tree in the campus grounds. Many suggestions were made to overcome the problem and finally relocation of the proposed department as an extension to the computer science building ensured the tree's safety and approval to build was granted. These negotiations had taken some months and, by November 1993, as building had not commenced, it was inconceivable that the department would be ready for occupation by autumn 1994. Temporary accommodation was required and it was decided, this time around, it would be provided in the chancellor's building with additional practical subject teaching space requirements satisfied by use of the sports hall. The university was characteristically vague about the detail of the layout and specificity of the proposed temporary accommodation. This, combined with the absence of the necessary work being undertaken to adapt the space to the school's requirements and the university's reluctance to keep the school informed of progress on the project, was not reassuring as the date for transfer had now been agreed and was rapidly approaching.

Keele University is campus-based and at the time of the school's transfer guaranteed student residential accommodation for two years of the three-year course. Students were offered campus accommodation for the first year, then tended to live out during the second year and return to campus for the final year. The organisation of the physiotherapy course was readily assimilated into this pattern, with second- and third-year students 'hot-bedding' their use of the accommodation as course arrangements alternated campus-based studies with clinical secondment.

Several issues with regard to the university accommodation available complicated negotiations. There were different levels of accommodation available with an associated scale of charges, whereas in NHS accommodation a single charge only operated. The academic year operated by the school was longer than that of the university with the second-year students having an accommodation requirement at each end of the university academic year. Undergraduates paid for the complete year for the accommodation selected, but second- and third-year physiotherapy students had been used to 'hot-bedding' as they alternated clinical and academic aspects of their course. This was more difficult to arrange due to the different charges appertaining to university accommodation. Due to the overshoot in numbers accepted for the 1993 intake, significantly more rooms were required for second-year students than the third year during campus-based components of the course. When second-year students were on placement, a substantial number of their rooms would remain empty during their secondment, although they remained responsible for continuing payment of rent. This was resolved by surrendering the hospital accommodation at Stoke-on-Trent and allowing second-year students to travel to placement in the Stoke-on-Trent hospitals from the university base. Finally, the accommodation facilities at the university were self-financing with significantly higher charges operating outside the defined university year.

After many meetings with Keele Hospitality to iron out the problems, agreement was finally reached in May. Students already undertaking the course had made their choices, hot-bedding arrangements were negotiated, lists of student names with dates were matched with accommodation availability and the list of students accepted for the 1994 course was promised for August, when it would be determined. All the arrangements and charges negotiated were confirmed by letter in May[20] and the head of department advised the region and the university of the satisfactory outcome of the protracted negotiations. It was considered this advance planning would assist the smooth transfer from the hospital to university environment and eliminate many of the concerns being voiced as the transfer date approached.

Transfer of the school's working base to a location approximately fifty miles distant from the RJAH posed particular problems for the principal's personal assistant (Elaina Evans) and secretary (Caroline Meeks) who for personal reasons were unable and/or unwilling to relocate to the university campus. There was no encouragement or incentive to facilitate their transfer and they sought alternative employment. The ideal solution to the dilemma was to ensure they were offered posts within the Oswestry area of equal salary and status to the ones they had occupied in the school. Eventually, Caroline found a post outside the NHS and Elaina was appointed to a different post within the trust. Jean Richards also decided not to transfer to the university and retired from her post when the Oswestry school base was closed.

June 1994 was a landmark month in the midst of all the activity surrounding the school's transfer. The first cohort to undertake the degree course successfully completed their studies and Marian Tidswell was awarded fellowship by the Chartered Society of Physiotherapy. The award is made to people recognised to have advanced the profession in specific areas and the citation accompanying the award identified two areas where this had been achieved. The first area recognised the development of the clinical education component of the course that had enhanced the development of clinical competence in the profession. The second area recognised her part in the development, implementation and support of the Certificate in Education course for the training of teachers of physiotherapy. The university was effusive in its recognition of the achievement and both professor Brian Fender (the vice chancellor) and Dr Slade (the director of academic affairs) wrote letters of congratulation to the recipient – in contrast to the WMRHA, NSHA and SHA, who made no comment.

Preparations for the removal continued without knowledge of the extent of campus accommodation that would be available; however, all equipment, furniture, records and staff and student course belongings were loaded into two extremely large furniture vans and set off for the journey to Keele. Once emptied, the rooms that had been occupied by the school since 1951 looked bleak and desolate. Barely had the furniture vans cleared the hospital grounds when the next occupants took up residence. Within an incredibly short time the school was converted to office accommodation and the Robert Jones and Agnes Hunt Orthopaedic and District NHS Trust established its operational base in the main corridor of the hospital, moving from its previously occupied office accommodation in the staff residency. Removal day marked the end of the school's eighty-five years of direct association with and dependence on a hospital base from which to operate. It was an emotional parting for some of the staff, but all faced the future with optimism.

NOTES

[1] Extracts from the minutes of the CSP Education Committee meeting, 8 May 1970

[2] *Working Paper 10, The National Health Service Community Care Act,* HMSO, 1990

[3] Extracts from the minutes of the ONSSP Policy Committee meeting, 5 December 1991

[4] Extracts from the minutes of the ONSSP Policy Committee meeting, 18 December 1991

[5] Extracts from the minutes of the ONSSP Policy Committee meeting, 5 December 1991

[6] Ibid

[7] Ibid

[8] *Guidelines for Written Submissions from Schools of Physiotherapy*, WMRHA Review of Physiotherapy Education and Training, 1992

[9] Extracts from the minutes of the ONSSP Management Board meeting, 16 June 1992

[10] Extracts from the minutes of the ONSSP Management Board meeting, 5 October 1992

[11] Ibid

[12] Extracts from the minutes of the ONSSP Management Board meeting, 17 August 1992

[13] Extracts from the minutes of the ONSSP Management Board meeting, 5 October 1992

[14] Extracts from the minutes of the ONSSP Management Board meeting, December 1992

[15] Extracts from the report by the principal to the awards ceremony, 12 November 1993

[16] Recommendations for rationalisation of physiotherapy education provision in the West Midlands region, 18 March 1993

[17] Extracts from the report by the principal to the awards ceremony, 12 November 1993

[18] Extracts from letter received from Alan Stedman, 29 March 1993

[19] Extracts from correspondence and telephone calls exchanged between the principal, Alan Walker, director of education at the CSP, Norma Brook, chair of the Physiotherapists Board of the CPSM and Sue Cox, WMRHA, between August and September 1993

[20] Letter from the accommodation services officer student accommodation centre of Keele University Hospitality, 6 May 1994

Chapter 18
A New Beginning

The physical transfer of the school to Keele University was negotiated over a period of months with particular emphasis on the position of the staff transferring from NHS to academic terms and conditions of service. During the negotiations, the university identified administration, teaching and research as the three core areas of academic endeavour on which staff grading requests were to be based. All university staff involved in grading negotiations had to demonstrate expertise in two out of these three areas to substantiate their case. Physiotherapy staff excelled in teaching and administration but, by virtue of the terms of NHS employment as teachers of physiotherapy, had little if any primary research experience. The university assured staff that this lack of research expertise and experience would not have a detrimental effect on the negotiations and indicated the department would have a grace period of five years in which to establish independent research from the university base. Despite assurances that staff would be fully assimilated within their first year on campus, they remained on the interim arrangements at the lowest possible points of the salary scales for more than three years. Between the start of negotiations and the arrival on campus, the university became focused on research as the main criterion for grading considerations and this delayed the full assimilation of the staff.

On removal day, ONSSP staff arrived ahead of the furniture vans to plan the most effective use of the temporary accommodation allocated pending completion of the purpose-built department. The designated space consisted of four offices or staff workrooms, two classrooms and a tutorial room located on the first floor of the chancellor's building at the centre of the campus, within easy walking distance of the dance studio in the sports centre where scheduled movement teaching would occur. The main problem encountered that day was that the planned alterations to the temporary accommodation had not been completed and the new department lacked telephone and computer network connections, rendering communication with other parts of the university or the outside world impossible.

Fortunately, owing to a puncture sustained en route by one of the furniture vans, they arrived later than scheduled and staff then spent the rest of the day transforming the empty spaces into effective working areas. The theory-dedicated classroom was of a suitable size to accommodate the complete student cohort, but the practical room was completely filled by the school's electrical equipment and plinths, and was too cramped for most teaching activities. Offices were allocated with the head of department and the examination officer occupying one of the two small rooms and senior teachers Marilyn Place and Maggie Bailey the other. The second largest room was nominated the departmental office and the largest room was used as a communal workroom for the seven remaining teaching staff. Each person was provided with a desk, computer and limited individual storage space. Movement equipment and plinths were stored in the dance studio in a room that could be adapted for theory or practical use with minimal effort. When all was in place, the vice chancellor, Professor Fender, met with staff for a small celebration to recognise his encouragement and support facilitating the development and implementation of the degree programme and the move to campus.

The move had been scheduled for the middle of the undergraduates' long summer break when the facilities were used extensively by delegates attending conferences and short courses throughout the vacation period. The venue for many of these events was the chancellor's building and removal day coincided with a high-profile conference for veterinary surgeons.

For the first week or so, until telephones were installed and connected, the only point of contact with university administration that staff were able to establish was through the reception desk on the ground floor of the chancellor's building. This was also the key point of contact for conference delegates and there were occasions when the two groups had minor interactions. It was not a very satisfactory arrangement as the move occurred the week following publication of the A-level results, always a busy time for the handling of enquiries from last-minute applicants and students offered places on the next course. Marilyn partially solved the problem by loaning her mobile phone to the department and this was in almost continuous use.

The morning following the move, staff found a number of university personnel eagerly waiting their arrival, seeking professional advice or treatment for a variety of conditions. The opportunity to gain ongoing support on campus rather than continuing with existing treatment programmes at the Stoke-on-Trent hospitals was a very attractive proposition to these individuals. As patient care was outwith the department's university brief, it was imperative to clarify its position and define its purpose without delay to avoid further confusion. On meeting with the registrar to discuss the matter, the head of department learned that physiotherapy had mistakenly been identified as a service department, which explained the arrival of potential patients earlier in the day. After lengthy and involved discussion, it was reconfirmed that the arrangements made prior to transfer identified physiotherapy as an academic department within the university, despite the lack of research in its academic profile. To clarify its purpose, it was named the department of physiotherapy studies.

Within days of the arrival on campus, an office manager was appointed who was conversant with the university's administrative structure and procedures. Her work was hampered by the fact that throughout the occupation of the chancellor's building, the department was not connected to the university's computer network. This meant it was excluded from the electronic messaging system on which the efficiency of the establishment depended. The first academic staff appointment made after the move was that of a half-time lecturer's post offered to a clinical therapist, Kryshia Dzeidzic, who was in the final stages of PhD studies while maintaining a full-time clinical post at Haywood Hospital. On successful completion of her studies she subsequently became a leading figure in the establishment of physiotherapy research across the West Midlands. Maintenance of the teaching schedule was aided by the recruitment of a former student, Ricky Mullis, to a lecturer's post on his completion of masters level studies in Manchester. Now that the department was university based, the obligatory teacher training required by the NHS was no longer necessary; however, Ricky undertook a comprehensive course offered by the university that prepared new lecturers for their role. Ricky effectively replaced Ken Stopani, who remained on long-term sick leave and subsequently left without ever taking up his university appointment. Nora Richards replaced him as examinations officer for the course until she decided to return to clinical work after little more than a year in the university environment.

Later, appointments of lecturer practitioners benefited all concerned by bringing dynamic clinical experts to the university to share their knowledge and enthusiasm with undergraduates. The final significant appointment made during this early period on campus was that of a dedicated clinical education coordinator. The appointee was Jenny Lowe, physiotherapy manager of the City General Hospital in Stoke-on-Trent and long-time clinical educator to students from the course. Management of the clinical education process was now more complicated, with additional hospitals being involved in the programme. Due to organisational change in the NHS, one of the more time-consuming tasks was the negotiation of annual contracts at each clinical base for the provision of placements. Jenny, an experienced physiotherapy manager well respected in both clinical and educational circles, brought experience and expertise to the negotiation of existing and additional placements required to enable the larger cohorts to complete a satisfactory clinical rotation.

Designation of the purpose of the department was the first of several matters that failed to transfer effectively from the negotiation table to the campus, as was discovered when students returned to continue their studies. Third-year students arrived first only to discover that no accommodation allocations had been made for them. Later, it was discovered that the book orders for all three years of the course had not been processed, despite the orders having been placed well within the university's time schedule. On further enquiry it appeared that the designation of the department, accommodation arrangements and book orders had not been processed appropriately as the university did not recognise the head of department and promptly disregarded any arrangements she made. This was a disappointing outcome to the many hours that had been spent negotiating arrangements to facilitate the students' transfer to campus; renegotiation was time-consuming and frustrating. Fortunately, all situations were ultimately resolved satisfactorily. By contrast, the academic staff of the university welcomed, supported and encouraged the new-comers. When all undergraduate cohorts had relocated to campus, they soon came to terms with their new teaching arrangements, and the second-year students were particularly grateful for the elimination of the long coach journey at each end of the university day.

Staff watched from a distance as their new building rapidly took shape and visited the site on two occasions to select their rooms and designate teaching areas. Plans had been made to accommodate a cohort of fifty-six when determining the appropriate size for theory and practical rooms. However, when the cost of the building was threatening to outstrip the finance available, room sizes were pared and the width of corridors reduced. Of major concern was that the theory room had now shrunk to the extent that it would no longer accommodate the full cohort; however, by a little rearrangement of the working area and the loss of a section of corridor, a room of appropriate size was constructed.

Well before Christmas of the first year on campus it was made known that the temporary accommodation in the chancellor's building was required for different users and there were also many complaints that the physiotherapy dominance of the dance studio was interfering with other undergraduate activities. The department was also keen to move to the new premises to enable connection with the university-wide computer network that had not been possible in the temporary accommodation. While remaining in the chancellor's building, physiotherapy studies was locked in an information vacuum. Taking account of the many pressures on the limited space available in the university, it was decided to advance the department's move to its new location and, in February 1995, it was installed on the middle floor of the new MacKay building.

The builders had been under great pressure to prepare the building for occupation in the shortest possible time; however, it seemed more important to vacate the chancellor's building and the dance studio than wait for building completion before the move. Only the middle floor of the building was habitable when the department moved to its new home. For the next two months, staff and undergraduates attempted to maintain their work schedules despite having moved to an active building site. All their activities were accompanied by hammering, drilling and workmen's voices necessarily raised to overcome the loud noise from radios permanently tuned to stations broadcasting frenetic programmes – a cacophony of sound that ate into the bones and sapped the energy. It was more difficult to cope with than had been major alterations to the hospital premises and, following the move, the department continued to operate in isolation, with no computer connections and surrounded by a lake of mud. Building work was completed by the middle of April. Over the Easter vacation, psychology moved to occupy the floor below the department and mathematics moved to the one above, thus enabling full appreciation of the excellent facilities now available.

The university was in the process of significant educational change around the time of the ONSSP's transfer to campus. The academic year structure had already been altered from three terms to two semesters, and now courses were to be modularised to enable standardisation of the volume of work across the three years of an individual course and to ensure academic parity between courses. The system introduced freedom and choice into a system that is often perceived as being inflexible.

The first cohort to graduate from the BSc (Hons) physiotherapy course operated by KU/ONSSP completed their studies in 1994, prior to the transfer of the school to the campus, and the course was validated for the qualification of a further four cohorts. Changes to the university's academic year had been assimilated into the existing course structure and, theoretically, no further significant change was required until course revalidation was required. However, the university encouraged existing courses to adopt modularisation prior to revalidation to standardise course presentation across the university in the shortest possible time.

When planning the initial degree course, the ONSSP was based in the NHS and compromises had been made in the distribution of subject teaching to accommodate the university's requirement for responsibility for twenty-five per cent of the academic input to the course. Now located on campus, the department of physiotherapy studies, formerly the ONSSP, was a recognised department of the university and chose to advance revalidation of the programme to accommodate the university's semester and modularisation requirements.

Marilyn had now completed masters-level studies in education and as course leader guided the development of the new degree programme during the academic year 1994–1995. Regular meetings were held with all subject leaders, clinical educators, the programmes office of the university and WMRHA representatives, and course planning progressed apace. Most participants contributed positively to the discussions but the department of biological science expressed concern about the concept and content of the physiology element of the course throughout the discussion period. The major change was that the majority of the teaching of physiology should revert to the department of physiotherapy studies personnel. It was proposed that the expertise of the biological sciences department would be utilised for practical and experimental work only in the revalidated degree course.

Significant effort had been applied over the previous decade to produce competent, committed autonomous practitioners by qualification and writing the course in a modular format enabled clarification of how this was achieved. In the new proposal, clinical education was renamed applied clinical science programme/fieldwork studies, and additional elements were introduced to encourage undergraduates to maximise their learning in this area of the course and to enable them to take some responsibility for shaping their individual learning experience. The overall aim of the course was to produce autonomous reflective practitioners, who were able to contribute to the evidence base of the profession.

To support undergraduate activity appropriately in the applied clinical science modules, a revised assessment form was required that was designed in a workshop attended by clinical educators, academic staff and students. The main categories of learning activity identified for assessment during the second year of the course were patient assessment, patient treatment, recording treatment and professional behaviour. Third-year students were additionally assessed on organisation and management. Each section was subdivided into constituent components that covered every aspect of the physiotherapist/patient interaction and was capable of being assessed in a dispassionate manner to exacting academic standards.

The new placement assessment system was piloted with second-year students as they embarked on the clinical education component of the course; it was found to be accurate and reliable, enabling effective evaluation of individual performance in each clinical location. All students were marked to the same objective criteria which also discriminated between closely matched performances that had proven to be inseparable with earlier evaluation systems. Following this piloting of the assessment form, it was accepted and incorporated into the degree documentation. The university accepted the objectivity and academic rigour of the process and commented that the department had proved the academic value of the clinical education experience.

The university rejected the first set of course documentation submitted, commenting that it was too cumbersome and contained more detail than was required by the university. As all the information presented was required for CPSM validation, a different presentation was considered and, over the Easter break, Kim Jones and Marilyn Place completely rewrote the submission. It was now divided into four documents: the course plan; course modules; educational justification; and appendices. This presentation was acceptable, the retrieval of specific information was easily achieved by all concerned and plans were made for validation of the course.

Initially, the completed documentation was circulated and reviewed by senior university personnel prior to an exploratory pre-validation meeting chaired by Dr Slade and attended by all concerned with the course development. The meeting was relatively informal and arranged to eliminate any outstanding problems that could interfere with the smooth running of the full validation event.

After a prolonged, detailed discussion of all aspects and elements of the proposed course the meeting was approaching conclusion when the head of the department of biological sciences raised very strong objections to the physiology content of the course. In his opinion the physiology component lacked the academic rigour the university required for an honours degree and was too selective, concentrating as it did on human physiology. A further half-hour of inconclusive discussion ensued before Dr Slade closed the meeting. He offered the department the choice of proceeding with validation of the submitted documentation or modifying the course to address the objections raised with resubmission of revised documentation at a later date. He stated that continuing to validation with the current documentation carried the risk of rejection by the validation panel, which would cause the department significant embarrassment in front of both the university and professional representatives.

After a short pause for reflection, the head of department stated that the course as presented satisfied all academic, professional and statutory requirements for successful validation and she considered that no useful purpose would be served by delaying the event. Dr Slade then decreed that further discussion be undertaken immediately with the biological science department to determine if a compromise could be reached. Two hours later it was obvious to the physiotherapists that the changes proposed by this department would be of significant detriment to the course and informed the departmental representative that validation was to proceed as arranged. Biological sciences asserted that the course would not receive a positive response to validation once the panel considered their objections. Marilyn and Marian met with Dr Slade to inform him of the unsuccessful outcome of the earlier discussion and were surprised to find that their decision was respected and the course proceeded to validation as planned.

Dr Slade chaired the validation event and Alan Walker, director of education from the CSP, and Norma Brook, chairman of the Physiotherapists' Board of the CPSM, represented the professional and statutory bodies. The course was presented to the first part of the meeting when members of the validation team had the opportunity to seek clarification or expansion of all aspects of the submission. All attendees were invited to make comment or raise concerns about the proposal, an ideal opportunity for the objections from the biological sciences department to be aired – but the opportunity was missed. As the meeting was drawing to a close, biological sciences belatedly raised their objections, but were informed that the meeting had moved on and they had missed the appropriate time on the agenda for such comments. Validation was successful with no alteration required to the presented documentation. Norma Brook agreed to be an external examiner to the new course, replacing Nigel Palastanga, who had completed his term of appointment.

Once validation was achieved, conversion courses were developed for the second and third year of the existing course to enable students who had commenced studies on the first degree course to be assimilated on to the new course from autumn 1995. This determined that the current third year became the second and last cohort to graduate in 1995 from the original degree course. From September 1995, for the first time in more than a decade, all undergraduates followed the same programme and staff were able to devote some time to the development of their own academic careers. During the academic year, staff were involved with lecturing on postgraduate and professional courses; they organised courses for the Chartered Physiotherapists in Education and presented at the WCPT conference in Washington DC. Kryshia completed her PhD and three other members of staff became actively involved in research, two enrolling for PhD studies. Another member of staff developed the first master's degree to be operated by the department. Several articles were published in scientific journals, three people contributed chapters to textbooks and another edited a textbook published during the year. Without exception, staff embraced the opportunities offered in the academic environment, justifying and consolidating the department's position on campus.

Forty-eight undergraduates commenced their studies in autumn 1995 of whom forty were supported by NHS bursaries and the remainder privately funded. Six of the privately funded candidates came from Norway, one from Greece and one from Canada. The course was now successfully established in the university environment, a fact that was reflected in the course report produced at the end of the 1995–1996 academic year.

External examiners commented positively on all aspects of the course and its administration, stating that the course content was applicable both professionally and academically, and compared favourably with professional courses of the same academic standard in other institutions.[1] Teaching and assessment was appropriate for the level of the course. However, staff were advised to continue development of the analytical approach in assessment not only to meet the academic requirements of an honours degree course but also to provide a sound foundation for the problem-solving skills required for effective patient care.[2]

First- and second-year students were generally very positive about their studies. The first year had started the new validated course and second-year students who had undertaken the first year on the previous course had coped well with the conversion course arranged for them, had enjoyed the second year and were well prepared for their third-year studies. The 1996 graduates were the first group to qualify from the new course and were significantly the least satisfied with the course. During their first year they had travelled from Oswestry two days a week to undertake their university studies. Following the move to campus at the end of their first year, they endured the ad hoc arrangements necessary while the department was housed in temporary accommodation prior to the move to the MacKay building. They piloted the new clinical assessment formats during the first year of their clinical education programme and then were given a conversion course to prepare them for completion of their studies on the new degree course. With so many changes occurring in the course's physical and academic environments during their three years of study, several commented that they felt like guinea pigs, and it is doubtful if they gained as much benefit from the university experience as did subsequent cohorts.

By the end of the 1995–1996 academic year, the department was firmly established within the university, with staff making significant progress in research and other academic activities required by the new environment. The main outstanding problem was the slow progress being made to assimilate staff to appropriate university grades.

Marian had completed her brief to establish the department in the university and it was now developing rapidly. All undergraduates now following the course had started their studies from the academic base. She retired from post, although she continued to work for the university for some time as deputy dean of the faculty of health, assisting members of the faculty to prepare masters courses in their various disciplines.

The department continues to thrive and is recognised as a leading programme for physiotherapy education and research in the academic environment as it had previously been in the NHS.

NOTES

[1] Extracts from the External Examiners Report in the 1995–1996 BSc (Hons) Course Report

[2] Ibid

Bibliography

Books

Barclay, Jean, *In Good Hands*, Oxford, Butterworth Heinemann Ltd, 1994

Berridge, John, *A Suitable Case for Treatment: A Case Study*, Milton Keynes, Open University Press, 1976

Carter, M., *Healing & Hope*, Robert Jones and Agnes Hunt Orthopaedic and District NHS Trust, 2000

Health Professions Order 2001, Statutory Instrument 2002 no. 254

Hunt, Dame Agnes, *This is My Life*, Edinburgh, Blackie, 1938

The Heritage of Oswestry – the Origin and Development of the Robert Jones and Agnes Hunt Orthopaedic Hospital, Oswestry, 1900–1975, Oswestry, The Robert Jones and Agnes Hunt Orthopaedic Hospital, 1975

Tidswell, M.E., *Orthopaedic Physiotherapy*, London, Mosby International Ltd, 1998

Tidswell, M., *Physiotherapy – A True Profession?*, unpublished MA Dissertation, 1991

Walton, J., ed., *The Oxford Companion to Medicine Vol. 2 N–Z*, Oxford, Oxford University Press, 1986

Wicksteed, J., *The Growth of a Profession*, London, Edward Arnold & Co., 1948

Young, P., *A Short History of the Chartered Society of Physiotherapy*, Chartered Society of Physiotherapy

Journals

Fairbank, J.C.T., J. Coupar, J.B. Davies and J. O'Brien, 'The Oswestry Low Back Pain Questionnaire', *Physiotherapy,* vol. 66, no. 8, pp. 271–273

Menzies, J.C., *Journal of the Old Oswestrian Physiotherapists Association*, 1956–1957

'100 years – 1894–1994' *Physiotherapy*, vol. 80, issue A

Supplement to *Newsletter,* July 1942, no. 11, British Orthopaedic Association,

'The Fire and After', *Orthopaedic Illustrated*, issue 12, winter 1971, p.11

Extracts of Minutes of Selected Meetings of:

Annual General Meetings of the Baschurch Convalescent Home

Annual Subscribers of the Baschurch Convalescent Home

Board of Management of the Robert Jones and Agnes Hunt Orthopaedic Hospital

Board of Management of the Shropshire Orthopaedic Hospital

Charted Society of Physiotherapy Education Committee

Committee of Visitors of the Shropshire Orthopaedic Hospital

Conference held at Shropshire Orthopaedic Hospital, 26 October 1931

Council of the Incorporated Society of Trained Masseuses

Examination Board of the Shropshire Orthopaedic Hospital

Executive Committee of the Baschurch Convalescent Home

General Committee of the Baschurch Convalescent Home

House Committee of the Shropshire Orthopaedic Hospital

Joint meeting between representatives of North Staffordshire and Shropshire Health Authorities, 8 July 1985

Management Committee of the Robert Jones and Agnes Hunt Orthopaedic Hospital

Medical Committee of the Shropshire Orthopaedic Hospital

ONSSP Education Committee

ONSSP Education Subcomittee

ONSSP Emergency Policy Committee Meeting, 27 July 1987

ONSSP Executive Education Committee

ONSSP School Management Board
ONSSP Policy Committee
Quarterly Meeting of the Baschurch Convalescent Home
RJAH Orthopaedic Hospital Management Committee
WMRHA Physiotherapy Training and Education Committee
WMRHA Regional Training Council

Correspondence

Accommodation Officer of Keele University to the Head of the Physiotherapy Department, 6 May 1994

Alan Stedman to the Principal, 29 March 1993

CPSM to ONSSP, 28 June 1989

CSP to ONSSP, 15 June 1988

CSP to ONSSP, 29 November 1988

CSP to Mrs Tidswell, 23 November 1987

NHS Executive to RHA, 17 February 1989

Slade, Dr E., to the principal of ONSSP, 30 November 1990

Spencer, R., to Mrs Tidswell, 29 June 1987

Talbot, D.F. to CSP Council, 5 February 1948

WMRHA RTO to the principal of ONSSP, 2 November 1988

Reports

Annual Reports of the Baschurch Convalescent Home

Beveridge, W., *Social Insurance and Allied Services*, CMD 604, HMSO, 1942

BSc (Hons) Course Report, July 1992

BSc (Hons) Course Report, August 1993

Clegg, *Report of the Standing Committee on Pay and Comparability of Paramedical Professions,* 1979

CPSM, *Administration and Financing of Schools of Physiotherapy,* 29 March 1973

CSP, *Clinical Training of Students at Schools of Physiotherapy*, 6 April 1973

CSP, *Inspection of Premises at Royal Salop Infirmary and Shropshire Orthopaedic Hospital,* 28 January 1932

CSP, *Revision of Arrangements for the Final Examination,* 2 March 1973

CSP Education Committee, *Shortage of Physiotherapy Teachers*, October 1975

External Examiners' Report contained in the BSc (Hons) Course Report, August 1996

Goodenough Report, *The Organisation and Future of Medical Education in the UK,* 1944

Graduate Diploma in Physiotherapy Course Report, September 1990

Graduate Diploma in Physiotherapy Course Report, November 1991

Graduate Diploma in Physiotherapy Course Report, December 1992

Graduate Diploma in Physiotherapy Course Report, August 1993

Guidelines for Written Submissions from Schools of Physiotherapy, WMRHA Review of Physiotherapy Education and Training, 1992

Halsbury, *Report of the Committee of Inquiry into the Pay and Related Conditions of Service of the Professions Supplementary to Medicine*, 1975

Houghton, *Report of the Committee of Inquiry into the Pay of Non-University Teachers*, December 1974

Principal's Report to the awards ceremony, 12 November 1993

Report of a meeting about the Physiotherapy Training School, 26 July 1949

Report of the CPSM Visit of Inspection, 17–18 April 1967

Report of the CPSM Inspection, 5–6 May 1981

Report of the CPSM Interim Inspection, 11–12 July 1983

Report of the Quinquennial CPSM Inspection, October 1986

Staff Development Group (Professional and Technical Staffs), *Physiotherapy Evaluation Group Report*, December 1987

WMRTC Staff Development Group (Professional and Technical Staffs) *Outcome of Visits to Schools of Physiotherapy in the West Midlands Region*, June 1987

WMRTC Staff Development Group (Professional and Technical Staffs) *Physiotherapy Manpower Needs – West Midlands Region*, Staff Development Group Report, June 1986

West Midlands Training Services (Training and Education Section), *Report on Physiotherapy Training in the West Midlands Region*, August 1988

Working for Patients – Education and Training in the NHS (further guidance), 1989

Working Paper 10, The National Health Service Community Care Act, HMSO, 1990

Personal memories

Abrahams, G., 1900–1988

Addie, I., 1939–1943

Alexander, A., 1943–1948

Anon – Set 33, 1970–1974

Gardner, M., 1943–1948

Linklater (née Knight), B., 1943–1948

Longson (née Taylor), E., 1923–1927

Lovatt, P., 1916–1919

Orritt, N., 1943–1948

Powell, M., 1936–1941

Roberts, H., 1943–1948

Rowe (née Bolton), K.E., 1936–1941

Student Memories 1959–1962

Taylor, F.M., 1914–1917

Index

A

ad hoc steering committee for clinical education, 229
advisor physiotherapists, 105
aftercare
 clinics, 56
 service, 56, 77
 sister, 54
Aguilar, Shân, 193, 215, 231, 237
Anderson, Margaret (Greta), 119, 128, 130, 131, 136, 143, 198
applied clinical science programme/fieldwork, 292
area management team (AMT), 155, 160
Arthur, Sister Hilda, 64
assistant physiotherapists, 104
associate membership of CSP, 77
Association of Orthopaedic Physiotherapists, 96
Association of Teachers of CSMMG, 55, 57
Aston Hall, 65, 86
Atkinson, Helen, 216, 232

B

Bailey, M, 277, 281
Bartlett, Miss, 81
Baschurch
 Convalescent Home, 29–30, 32–40
 Convalescent Home and Hospital, 35
 School of Massage, 43
 Shropshire, 19
Beardwell, Martin, 205, 214, 224, 230, 234
Bebb, Judy, 194, 231
Bell, Matron, 70, 97
Bentley, Joyce, 111
Beveridge Report, 73
Birchenough, Miss, 130
Birmingham
 Regional Health Board, 137
 Regional Hospital Board, 88
 University, 62, 272, 274
Blair, George, 273
Bloor, Steve, 233, 234, 249, 252
Board of Management, 74, 77, 78
Bond, Chris, 217
Border Counties Advertiser, 89
Boreatton
 Hall, 25, 46
 Park, 23, 33
Bottomley, Virginia, 273
Bourne, Jean, 238, 243
Braid, Gordon, UGM Northern Unit SHA, 205–7, 213, 229–31, 233, 237, 241, 270, 273
Bright, Karen, 193, 238
British Medical Journal, 28
British Orthopaedic Association, 114
Brodie, Dr, 202
Bromley, Ida, 185
Brook, Norma, 295
Bury, Major Lindsay, 79, 98

C

Caney, Doreen, 210
Cannell, Winifred (Wyn), 119, 128, 135, 137, 146, 155, 161, 163, 198
CARB, 151
Cash, Joan, 118
Central Council for the Care of Cripples, 114
Certificate in Education (Further Education), 159, 284
Challinor, Mr P.J., 118, 121
chancellor's building, Keele University, 257, 281, 286
Chanmugan, Mrs, 135, 136
Chartered Society of Massage and Medical Gymnastics (CSMMG), 49, 60, 61, 74, 92
Chartered Society of Physiotherapy, ix, 75, 77, 78, 79, 93, 119, 141, 148, 273, 279
Chester College, 177, 250
City General Hospital, 132, 133, 135
Clegg Report, 154
Colbert, Mr W., 130
Conjoint Examination (CSMMG), 49, 55, 87, 89 (Oswestry), 49
Cooke, Miss P.M., 55
Copthorne Hospital, 108, 109
Council for Professions Supplementary to Medicine (CPSM), 111, 147, 280
Council of the CSP, 87
course planning and review committee, 229
Coventry School of Physiotherapy, 220, 224, 249, 274
Cox, Sue, 273, 277
CPSM/CSP inspection, 119, 122, 123, 163, 169, 183, 206
Crewe and Alsager College, 250
Crowe, Mr, 130
Cruttenden, Mr D., 130
CSP director of education, 250
CSP inspection, 95, 108, 110

D

Dalton, Miss, 55, 66, 70, 78, 96
dance studio, 286, 287
Davies, Jean, 164, 174, 181, 182, 190
department of biological science, 292
Department of Health, 113
department of physiotherapy studies, 288, 292
departmental superintendent, 104
Derwen Cripples Training College, 56, 86, 87, 109
District Health Authority, 187
Dobny, Dr, 119
Dzeidzic, Kryshia, 288, 295

E

Education Committee of the CSP, 123, 199
Elder, Miss, 95
electric treatment room, 84
electrotherapy, 59, 78–80
Elphick, Miss, 119
Emergency Medical Service, 68
Ennals, David, 153
Evans, Elaina, 238, 283
Evans, Miss Sybil, 110, 119
Ewart, Miss, 54
external examiners, 262, 264, 296

F

Faculty of Physiotherapy, 39
Fender, Professor Brian, 284, 287
Field, Jane, 44
Final examination, 76, 81, 110
First World War, 45
Fletcher, Mr, 200
Fletcher-Cook, Phyl, 182, 190, 199
Florence House, 29
Fowler, Lt J.A. (Tony), 156, 162, 164
Frith, Eileen, 242

G

Gifford, Mr, 95
Gittings, Kevin, 250
Glasgow Royal Infirmary, 66
Goff, Barbara (Bobbie), 102, 114, 124, 128, 136, 139, 156, 164, 179, 180, 185, 190
Goodenough Report, 75
Goodford, Emily, 20, 27–30, 33, 37, 50
Goss, Else, 182
Graduate Diploma in Physiotherapy, 232
Grant, Margaret, 191
Graveling, Madge, 118
Gredington Children's Annexe, 64
Gwynne, Mrs, 129, 130

H

Halsbury Report, 146, 152, 155
Harrison Hut, 128, 134, 137, 139
Harrison, Mrs, 130
Hart, Dr, 150
Hawley, Miss, 110
Hayden, Decima (Jake), 44
Hayden, Dorothy, 44
Haywood Hospital, 174, 239
HC7733, 158, 180
Health Professions Council, 111
Heywood, Tony, 205
Holbourn, Philip, 202, 234
Holden, Penny, 138
Hollins, Barbara, 243
Hollis, Margaret, 195
Holmes, Jane, 215, 231, 237
Hopkins, Sue, 191
hospital fête, 157
Hospital Management Committee, 88, 96, 98, 102, 103, 104, 105, 108, 112, 117, 120, 122
Hothersall, Dr, 150
Houghton Committee Report, 152
Howl, Miss, 94
Humphreys, Jill, 183, 184
Hunt
   Agnes Gwendoline, 19, 23, 27, 32, 33, 37, 45, 50, 56, 68, 70, 77, 86, 88
   Florence Marianne, 22, 25, 28, 31, 44, 45
   Rowland, 34
   Rowland, 1829–1879, 22, 25

I

Incorporated Society of Trained Masseuses (ISTMS), 28, 39, 40, 43, 46, 47, 48, 49, 92
Institute of Massage and Remedial Gymnastics, 49
Institute of Orthopaedics, 280
Intermediate examination, 76, 99

J

Jahn, Eva, 236
Jean Davies Memorial Prize, 194, 242
Jeffers, Ruby, 183
John, Elsa, 80, 88, 93, 95, 105, 115, 123
Johnson, Dr, 122
joint superintendents, 33, 42
Joint Validation and Recognition Panel, 234, 250
Jones, Beris, 154
Jones, Kim, 237, 293
Jones, Robert, 34, 35, 36
Jones, Ron, 217
Jordan, Rachel, 124

K

Kay, Ralph, 135, 154, 156, 164, 179
Keele University, 229, 250, 272, 273, 282
Kempster, Miss, 116
Kenyon, Eliza, 30
Kenyon, Lord, 65, 69
Kidd, Diana, 111, 115, 117

L

Lackenau, Dr, 80
lady pupil nurse, 26, 38
Langshaw Rowland, Mrs, 118, 122
Lavall, Mr, 60
League of Friends of the RJAH, 173
Limes, the, 137, 160, 168
Liverpool University Medical School, 62, 63, 67, 140
Lloyd, Dr, 110
Lloyd, Polly, 30
London Hospital, 28, 63
Longson, Edna, 53
Lowe, Jenny, 289
Lowndes, Mr, 130
Lymn, Janet, 160, 174, 193
Lythgoe, Mr T., 118

M

MacKay building, 291
MacKenzie, Kirk, 270
Maitland, Geoffrey, 123
Manchester Royal Infirmary, 62
Manley Memorial Prize, 138
Manley, Elizabeth Anne, 28
Market Drayton chest clinic, 109
Marriot, Miss, 82
massage, 39
massage department, 53
Maude, Archdeacon, 30
McSweeney, Mr T., 122
Medical Advisory Committee, 105, 111, 122, 217, 222
medical electricity, 46, 48
and light therapy, 58, 61
medical rubbing, 28, 40
medical school, Birmingham University, 62
Meeks, Caroline, 238, 283
membership of the Chartered Society of Massage and Medical Gymnastics, 55
membership of the Chartered Society of Physiotherapy, 75
Middlesbrough, 27
midwife, 27
Minister of Health, 74, 153
Ministry of Health, 114, 119, 120
Mockett, Simon, 262
Mogg, Phil, 218, 224
Moore, Dr, 200, 205

Morda Hospital, 109, 116
MSc in Habilitation, 191
Mullis, Ricky, 289
Multidisciplinary Team, 202, 203
Murray, Miss Evelyn, 55, 64, 70, 78, 98
Myles, Professor Sandra, 262

N

National Health Service, 66, 73, 74, 95, 187
National Organisation for Physiotherapy Students, 157
National Union for Students, 157, 251
Neill, Ann, 190, 231
North Staffordshire Area Health Authority (NSAHA), 147, 159
North Staffordshire Health Authority (NSHA), 196, 200, 215, 219, 230, 252, 270, 271
North Staffordshire Royal Infirmary, 122, 132, 133
Northern Guild, 39
northern sector SAHA, 147
northern unit SHA, 204, 237, 252
NSHA School of Nursing and Midwifery, 276
nursing subcommittee, 101, 105, 109, 121

O

O'Connor, Professor Brian, 150
Objective Structured Clinical Examination (OSCE), 201
Objective Structured Practical Examination (OSPE), 243, 260
Old Oswestrian Physiotherapists Association, 101
Ollerton, 27, 29
ONSSP Education Committee, 129, 141, 155, 160, 163, 187, 192, 270
ONSSP Executive Committee, 200, 201, 203
ONSSP Management Board, 270
ONSSP Policy Committee, 218, 229, 232, 236, 249, 270
OOPA, 101, 138
Orme, Miss, 128
Orthopaedic Nursing Certificate, 38, 57, 62, 81, 123, 139
Orthotic Research and Locomotor Assessment Unit, 182, 260
Oswestry and District Hospital, 102, 109
Oswestry and North Staffordshire School of Physiotherapy, 129, 211, 218, 221, 223, 224, 249–53, 274, 275
Oswestry League of Nurses, 101, 102
Oswestry Low Back Pain Disability Questionnaire, 182
Oswestry School of Massage and Medical Gymnastics, 77
Oswestry/Wolverhampton School of Physiotherapy, 93, 102
Owtram, Miss, 82, 93

P

Paget, Rosalind, 28
Palastanga, Nigel, 236, 254, 262, 295

Palmer, Margaret Dora, 28
Park Hall
   camp, 85
   Military Hospital, 50
Parry, Ron, 270, 274
Part 1 examination, 149
Part 2 examination, 149
pathology department, 112, 120
PCAS, 241
Pearce, E.C., 47, 54
Penicillin, 67
Philbrook, Sheila, 225
physiotherapy department, 84
Physiotherapy Evaluation Group, 210, 211, 212, 213, 216, 222, 279
Place, Marilyn, 192, 238, 281, 292
Powell, Mary, 63, 64, 66, 99, 101, 113, 118, 121, 130, 195, 225
Preliminary examination, 76, 103
probationer nurse, 26

Q

Queen Elizabeth Hospital School of Physiotherapy, 221, 224, 249, 274
Queens Nurse, 27
Queens Square, 114

R

Red Cross, 50
registered nurse training, 38
Rhodes, Susan, 137
Richards, Jean, 191, 199, 231, 235, 240, 283
Richards, Nora, 180, 191, 231, 289
Roaf, Mr, 114, 118, 121
Robert Jones and Agnes Hunt Orthopaedic Hospital, 73, 81, 92
Roberts, Hazel, 89, 90
Robertson, Sandy, 281
Robinson, Lucy Marianne, 28
Robinson, Mrs, 130
Rogers, Jean, 96, 98, 117, 119, 128, 136, 155, 157, 164, 179, 180, 183, 185, 186, 190, 231
Rose, Cath, 182, 190, 225, 234, 235, 243
Rose, Mr G.K., 118
Rowlands, Sister Mary, 69, 90, 113
Royal Alexandra Hospital, Rhyl, 27, 33
Royal Charter, 49, 110
Royal Hospital, Wolverhampton, 81, 89, 92, 93
Royal Orthopaedic Hospital School of Physiotherapy, 224, 249, 274
Royal Southern Hospital, Liverpool, 59
Ruabon Hills, 67
Rushden, 27
Rutherford, Ian, 277

S

Salop Area Health Authority (SAHA), 147, 162, 171, 173
Salop Area Management Team, 173, 175
Salop Infirmary, 27, 29
Sankey, Avis, 99
Savin, Ann, 119, 128
school badge, 130
school of Physical Education and Recreation, 202, 229
Second World War, 65–70

Selattyn, 68
seminar rooms, 176, 206, 225
Sex Discrimination Act 1975, 161
Shotton, B, 151
Shrewsbury Hospital Management Committee, 108
Shropshire Health Authority, 196, 215, 230, 270, 271
Shropshire Orthopaedic Hospital, 50, 65
Shropshire War Memorial Societies, 50
Silk, Jeff, 148, 172, 204
Slade, Dr E., 251, 275, 277, 284, 293, 294, 295
Slee, Mr, 124, 129
Society of Trained Masseuses, 28
spinal disorders unit, 182
sponsored disco, 174, 185
St Thomas' Hospital, London, 66
Staff Development Group, 210, 211, 212
staff/student liaison committee, 270
Stedman, Alan, 273, 274, 275
Steele, Anne, 164
Stockbridge, John, 217
Stoke-on-Trent HMC, 121, 128, 137
Stopani, Ken, 190, 197, 199, 202, 234, 238, 250, 253, 255, 277, 281, 289
Summerhays, Miss, 93
sunlight department, 53
Swedish remedial exercise, 40, 42
Swedish remedial gymnast, 45

T

Talbot, Dorothy, 70, 80, 81, 87, 88, 93, 96, 103, 104, 116, 117, 121, 122
Taylor, Dr, 79
Thorpe, Miss, 93
Tidswell, Marian, 135, 136, 155, 159, 168, 174, 179, 196, 198, 202, 204, 210, 216, 234, 238, 242, 277, 278, 283, 297
Tudor, Mrs, 104, 111
tuition fees, 47
TUPE, 276, 281
typhoid, 89–91

U

UCCA, 241
University of Keele Selected Ordinances, Regulations and Examination Information, 265

V

VAD nurses, 45
Validation & Recognition Panel, 234, 235, 250
Vernon, Heather, 245

W

Walker, Alan, 250, 295
Walker, Mr, 130
Ward, Dr Donald, 124, 129, 150
Watson-Jones, Sir Reginald, 101
Webb, Jean, 183, 184
West London Hospital, Hammersmith, 27
West Midlands College of Physiotherapy, 221

West Midlands Regional Health Authority, 217, 251, 269, 271, 280
West Midlands Regional Physiotherapy Training and Education Committee, 224, 226, 249, 270
West Midlands Regional Training Council, 210, 217, 249, 275
West Midlands regional training officer, 218, 224
West Midlands Regional Training Services Report, August 1988, 223
West Midlands SDG PEG interim statement, June 1987, 214, 219, 279
West Midlands SDG PEG Report, December 1987, 219–21
West Midlands SDG Report, 211, 212
Whitley Council (PTA), 151
Wingfield Morris Orthopaedic Hospital, 113
Wolverhampton Group HMC, 103
Wolverhampton Polytechnic, 250
Wolverhampton School of Physiotherapy, 218, 224, 249, 274, 280
Wood, Dorothy, 44
Wood, Pat, 154, 164, 182
Woods, Leanne, 231, 238
Working Paper 10, 251, 269, 270
Wrexham Accident Hospital, 103
Wrexham Maelor Hospital, 103

Printed in Great Britain by
Amazon.co.uk, Ltd.,
Marston Gate.